NEW WAYS OF

UNDERSTANDING

AUTISM

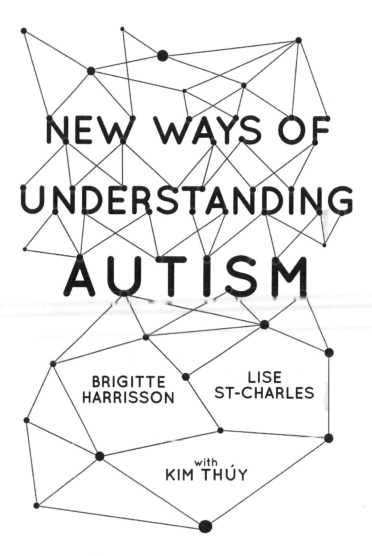

NEW WAYS OF
UNDERSTANDING
AUTISM

**BRIGITTE
HARRISSON**

**LISE
ST-CHARLES**

with
KIM THÚY

Translated by Juliet Sutcliffe

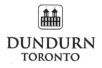

DUNDURN
TORONTO

Printer: Webcom, a division of Marquis Book Printing Inc.
Cover concept: Stefano Pietramala (STUDIO IANUS, Milan)

Library and Archives Canada Cataloguing in Publication

Title: New ways of understanding autism / Brigitte Harrisson, Lise St-Charles, with Kim Thúy;
translated by Juliet Sutcliffe.
Other titles: Autisme expliqué aux non-autistes. English Names: Harrisson, Brigitte, 1961- author. |
St-Charles, Lise, 1957- author. | Thúy, Kim, author.
Description: Translation of: L'autisme expliqué aux non-autistes. | Includes bibliographical references.
Identifiers: Canadiana (print) 20189068701 | Canadiana (ebook) 2018906871X | ISBN
9781459743601 (softcover) | ISBN 9781459743618 (PDF) | ISBN 9781459743625 (EPUB)
Subjects: LCSH: Autism spectrum disorders—Miscellanea.
Classification: LCC RC553.A88 H37213 2019 | DDC 616.85/882—dc23

1 2 3 4 5   23 22   21 20 19

This translation was made possible by the financial support of **Société de développement des
enterprises culturelles (SODEC).** We also acknowledge the support of the **Canada Council for
the Arts,** which last year invested $153 million to bring the arts to Canadians throughout the
country, and the **Ontario Arts Council** for our publishing program. In addition, we acknowledge
the financial support of the **Government of Ontario,** through the **Ontario Book Publishing Tax
Credit** and **Ontario Creates,** and the **Government of Canada.**

Nous remercions le **Conseil des arts du Canada** de son soutien. L'an dernier, le Conseil a investi
153 millions de dollars pour mettre de l'art dans la vie des Canadiennes et des Canadiens de
tout le pays.

Care has been taken to trace the ownership of copyright material used in this book. The authors
and the publisher welcome any information enabling them to rectify any references or credits in
subsequent editions.

— J. Kirk Howard, President

The publisher is not responsible for websites or their content unless they are owned by the publisher.

Printed and bound in Canada.

VISIT US AT

dundurn.com | @dundurnpress | dundurnpress | dundurnpress

Dundurn
3 Church Street, Suite 500
Toronto, Ontario, Canada
M5E 1M2

A Note on Language

THE LANGUAGE SURROUNDING autism is currently in flux. Until recently, "person first language" was in general use — "a person with autism" was preferred. The standard usage has been changing, however, as people with autism increasingly join the conversation. In *New Ways of Understanding Autism*, identification-first language is used — "an autistic person" — as it is becoming increasingly prevalent. Autistic people who prefer the term often explain their choice thus: autism is not something I have; autism is an integral part of who I am. Although a decision has been made on appropriate usage for this book, autistic people should always be consulted about how they would prefer to be addressed.

Contents

Introduction

PEOPLE ARE CONSTANTLY asking questions about autism. How does an autistic person perceive the world? Why does she make all those movements? How does he feel? Is he all right? These questions come up all the time, and answers are often offered by people who aren't aware of current developments in autism research in the scientific literature. So what are the answers?

This book aims to present clearly the directions suggested by recent discoveries and theories, combining knowledge of autistic functioning and a new understanding of what it means to treat autism. Descriptions are written from the perspective of an autistic person, to allow neurotypical readers a basis for comparison with their own experience. Until now, most writing on autistic function has been based on a neurotypical person's viewpoint, which led to an analysis that did not give a logical and coherent picture of autism. In this book, we bring together the lived

Brigitte: I remember a time when I was all alone, struggling to do what people told me to do, never enjoying life because everything I did was what others had asked of me. I could never be myself. I could never value myself as an individual because I was surrounded by neurotypical people who did the same things as I did, but for different reasons. I had a key ring that read "Just visiting this planet." And that was my reality. I did things for other people. I could never do anything for me. The outside world guided my life. I wasn't in my own little world, but stuck, with my autistic brain oriented outward. I ate because it was lunchtime. My showers lasted seven minutes thirty-three seconds. And so on. Life had no meaning.

experience of autistic people, real-life stories from parents, and suggested therapeutic approaches to show readers that there is hope for autistic people.

These approaches to interpretation and treatment come mainly from *Fonctionnement interne de la structure de la pensée autistique* (Harrisson 1993),[*] whose description of autistic function corresponds to recent work in the field and demonstrated results in the scientific literature. Since it was developed in the 1990s, this theory of autism has been presented to thousands of people and has stood the test of time. It's a way of understanding autism that proposes treatment suited to addressing neurodevelopmental disruption and the people who are affected by it. Using this theory, we created the SACCADE model and SACCADE Conceptual Language

---

[*] Not published in English translation. Roughly, the title means "the internal structure of autistic thought."

> *Lise:* Analyzing behaviour from one's own frame of reference is always tricky. If you don't know the frame of reference of another person or of a particular community, you can make big mistakes. One day I was in a conference room in a hotel. In the room opposite, some Japanese tourists were burping loudly during their meal. The people I was with were quick to remark on the rudeness of these tourists. I had to explain to them that in Japan, people do this to show satisfaction after a meal. In a Quebec context, the noises were perceived as a lack of manners, whereas in Japan they are valued!

(SCL),* which are helping autistic people communicate. Just as sign language was developed by deaf people and Braille by a blind man, SCL was created by an autistic person.

The needs of autistic people are almost always interpreted in the same way — from a neurotypical viewpoint. We analyze and treat each need separately, without any consistent reference to the autistic function described in the literature. For example, if an autistic person presents with a severe sensory sensitivity, we often try to increase sensory stimulation to help her get used to it. But we should instead understand that she is behaving this way because she's at a particular developmental stage; she is standing in front of a door that she can't open, so she can't move on to the next developmental stage.

---

* SACCADE is an intervention model conceived in Quebec by the authors. SACCADE is an acronym for Structure et Apprentissage Conceptuel Continu Adapté au Développement Évolutif, which translates roughly as "continuous conceptual learning aimed at producing progressive development."

Autism is a wiring and connections issue. Neurotypical individuals are not yet accustomed to taking the overall autistic framework into account when they seek to understand autistic needs and behaviours.

We felt it was important to bring together three points of view in this book: those of the autistic person, the parent, and the experienced professional. We saw these three perspectives as essential for an overview of the topic. We believe that these different interest groups should talk to each other, without any one being seen as lesser. We would like to do away with the situation in the field today, which is like a tower of Babel. There's inconsistency, lack of improvement, increased costs to society, saturation of services, wasted lives, professional disappointments, and above all, the transformation of autistic people into lab rats and currency to be traded, which punishes them instead of helping them. Everyone with a stake in the field of autism pays the price for this, and yet the situation could be very different.

Intervention is a deeply complex task, given that autism is a neurodevelopmental disorder — a cerebral wiring issue that affects development. Every attempt at treatment may affect brain plasticity. Everyone involved with autistic people, then, needs to work together so that the intervention makes sense for each individual. The person's needs must be monitored so that we avoid implementing prolonged therapeutic practices without knowing what effects they will have. Unfortunately, in this field, we still don't fully understand what a sensible treatment program looks like. Because only a few guiding principles exist, because autism "specialists" are popping up like mushrooms, and because parents can shop around for autism treatments, it's difficult to get a true picture of the needs associated with autism. How can we expect parents to become experts in the most complicated neurodevelopmental disorder there is, when even the professionals haven't fully understood it?

We are hoping with this book to turn a page in the history of autism and move to a new understanding of it — one that focuses on putting the needs of the autistic person where they should be: at the centre.

1

Toward a Unifying Explanation of Autism

THE PICTURE THAT SCIENCE paints of autism has changed radically over the past few years. But to fully understand these new discoveries, we need to be able to combine them with the lived experience of autistic people — an aim that science is gradually working toward.

We owe the description of classic autism to the Austrian psychiatrist Leo Kanner, who, in 1943, described autistic people as having two characteristics: aloneness (extreme solitude) and sameness (immutability, a desire to maintain permanence). The word "autism" had first been used in 1911, by Swiss psychiatrist Eugen Bleuler: it comes from the Greek word *autos*, meaning "self." According to Kanner, autism was an "innate" disorder.

In the 1980s, the British psychiatrist Lorna Wing proposed a definition of autism based on a trio of areas affected in autistic people: communication, interaction and stereotyped behaviour, and restricted interests.

In 2013, the fifth edition of the *Diagnostic and Statistical Manual of Mental Disorders* (*DSM*), published by the American Psychiatric Association, established the following criteria to create a consistent international standard:

- "persistent deficits in social communication and social interaction"
- "restricted, repetitive patterns of behavior, interests, or activities"
- symptoms that show up early in life
- symptoms that cause significant difficulties for daily life

None of these traditional descriptions of seemingly antisocial or bizarre behaviours takes into account the point of view of an autistic person. We therefore needed a new perspective: an overview of the theoretical descriptions that also incorporates both the lived experience of the autistic individual and a broad range of professional expertise with the aim of adopting an entirely new vision of autism.

The predictions we made from this approach were borne out in practice. They allowed us to make sense of theories that had stood up for more than thirty years. But the classic definition and the proposed reframing rely on totally opposite aspects of physical reality. According to the French sociologist Brigitte Chamak, when autistic people talk about autism, they aren't talking about the same things as neurotypical people. Most people discuss the specifics of perception, how information and emotions are dealt with. The most intuitive description given is, without a doubt, Temple Grandin's. Grandin is an autistic American, a well-known professor of animal science. According to her, autistic people are visual thinkers.

Until the emergence of neuroscience and a more precise understanding of development (for example in babies), it was generally believed that we could acquire a comprehensive understanding of internal human function by observation — that observers would understand autistic people by watching their behaviour. However, the discoveries of recent years and the actual experiences of autistic people, including Temple Grandin and Brigitte Harrisson, indicate that this is not the case. The naive, popular concept of autism is incompatible with research in neuroscience and child development, as well as with the lived experience of autistic individuals.

In order to move beyond simplistic and compartmentalized ideas of autism, we consider the fact that several very different theories can explain a single phenomenon and all be equally valid. And if two theories interpret the same phenomenon, the observer will choose the one that suits him or her best. So people's understandings of autism will differ based on their vision, role, and knowledge.

Throughout the history of autism, we have seen the emergence of models or theories of increasing quality, from Kanner to current neuroscience, via Simon Baron-Cohen's theory of mind, Uta Frith's concept of weak central coherence, and Sally Ozonoff's notion of executive (dys)function. Because each of these models contains an important piece of the puzzle, it's possible that we might one day come up with a broad theory of autism, one that will take into account all the developmental stages of the autistic brain and have predictive capacity. Even if we aren't there yet, we do already have a coherent theory: the hypothesis of the internal function of autistic thought structure (Harrisson and St-Charles). We believe this is the only hypothesis that draws together all the necessary explanations in order to offer an overall description of autism; it therefore forms the basis of our reflections here. This is not, strictly speaking, a scientific theory, but rather a theory whose principles and observed phenomena are confirmed in current scientific research. Our theory of autism takes into account scientific literature, recent discoveries, treatment methods, and lived autistic experience. Our clinical approach has been effective for over ten years, regardless of the age of the autistic person, the extent to which he or she is affected, and whether or not other problems are also present. It also has a certain amount of predictive power.

More and more people know of the existence of autism spectrum disorder (ASD), which incorporates what were previously known as Asperger's syndrome and classic autism. But knowing it exists doesn't necessarily mean understanding what it actually is. We believe that the images currently associated with autism tend toward catastrophic scenarios.

People often describe autism in three main ways. They tell us that autism is a plague, an epidemic. They talk about bizarre behaviour and autistic meltdowns in a way that evokes outdated beliefs: autistic people are children off in their own worlds, banging their heads against a wall, never having relationships with others, but possibly gifted with exceptional talents. Finally, society condemns people to their autism before they have a chance to develop: they are thought to be unable to achieve independence, so people jump in to plan their lives and organize their future security.

Another phenomenon clouds the picture further. The media often emphasizes autistic meltdowns, as well as the Rain Man–like behaviour and abilities of some autistic people (who actually represent around 1 percent of those on the autism spectrum). Any autistic people who don't have these traits then become non-autistic, or merely uninteresting, in the popular imagination. Worse still, if people can't "see" autism, they don't take it seriously.

Certain persistent autism taboos, along with the effects of stigmatization, might be the origin of two survival phenomena among friends and family of an autistic person, the "collateral carriers" of autism: either they rush to hide autistic behaviour to make the person's condition invisible or, paralyzed with fear, they do nothing at all, which wastes precious time for the autistic person.

Such beliefs, of course, perpetuate a perception of autism as something to fear, and lead to unhealthy behaviour: instead of interacting with the autistic person, we talk to the people around them. This means others speak for the autistic person. We talk a lot about autism itself, about the suffering of parents and families, the challenges facing professionals, but we don't talk enough about autistic people themselves. We don't hear autistic voices.

Autistic people are condemned to live in a parallel world because those around them don't understand their condition and can't meet their needs. However, this parallel world exists and must be charted. Just as the first explorers developed maps of the world, so we need to map the autistic brain. Until we have a complete map of the connections in the brain, and until we understand its workings and the physiological effects of the way the autistic brain is configured, we won't be able to give a complete definition of autism. Moreover, even if the pictures we obtain from magnetic resonance imaging establish the link between brain wiring and physical function, they will never be able to describe the real impact of the autistic brain on the everyday lives of autistic people. We must therefore take into consideration the explanations and descriptions of the people concerned: autistic people themselves. We can no longer act as if they are unable to speak for themselves.

Parents are exhausted, overloaded with unclear responsibilities, and bitter that they don't see more improvement in their child after significant effort and many specialist interventions. They feel powerless in the face of autism, whether their child is severely affected or has graduated from university. They're convinced they must have missed something. However, some autism studies now recommend trusting the parents' instincts.

As a society, we rarely put the experience of seasoned autism professionals to good use. This is a serious mistake, because it takes dozens of years of intervention, training, and teaching to come to an understanding of what works and what has never worked, the origins of certain practices, and the mistakes practitioners keep repeating. Professionals have lived through their own difficult experiences, and a rapid turnover of specialists is not uncommon. Indeed, autism treatment may decline in quantity and in quality because fewer and fewer experienced practitioners are working in the field.

The history of autism helps us to understand how we have reached this point, why no treatment seems to work, and how far we've gone off course over the last seventy years. We've spent a long time moving from observing autistic behaviour to gaining biological knowledge.

In the 1950s, people used to believe that autism was the parents' fault, that they had caused their child to be "functionally handicapped." But at the beginning of the 1960s, the American TEACCH (Treatment and Education of Autistic and Related Communication Handicapped Children) team directed by psychologist Eric Schopler destroyed this theory by positing that autism was a biological difference and that autistic children were "educable." The TEACCH program's massive success proved him right.

Then it was suggested that autism was a socialization disorder, a myth that persists today in spite of advances in neuroscience. However, in 1989, the German psychologist Uta Frith proposed that autism is a result of weak central coherence (having difficulty combining single elements into a meaningful whole). Autistic people have trouble reading social situations; socialization difficulties are therefore a secondary effect of autism.

Some researchers have also maintained that autism is a behavioural disorder. This myth still lingers because we don't yet know how to distinguish behaviour resulting from autistic brains from behaviour that could be classified as wilfully bad. This understanding of autism as developmental doesn't take into account Ozonoff's theory of executive function (the mental processes that allow conscious control of thought and actions). In 1991 the difficulties involved in planning, mental flexibility, and organization became more widely known, showing that certain behavioural problems have nothing to do with wilfulness on the part of the autistic person.

During the 1980s, we were able to kill off another myth, the one that claimed autism was an attachment disorder. The studies are clear on this point: autistic people do form attachments. Moreover, researcher Simon Baron-Cohen used his theory of mind and social intelligence to explain some of the mental processes of autism: it's not an attachment disorder, but rather a different concept of self and other. The theory of mind suggests that autistic people are unable to figure out other people's mental states. Neurotypical mental processes allow people to adjust their behaviour to that of others by using mental images of themselves and others. Some autistic people are unable to do this. Sometimes they don't know that the person in front of them has thoughts different from their own. The theory of social intelligence is that autistic people are unable to visually decode the social meaning of other people's emotions. So an autistic person might see someone frown and understand that the other person is angry. But if that person is frowning because they are looking at a sunny landscape, the autistic person will still see anger, because his or her reading of the other person is based on learned information and not on a detected emotion.

More recently, autism was thought to be an emotional disorder or even that it prevented emotion. The Portuguese neurologist Antonio Damasio has been writing since 1996 about "the feeling of what happens." This led to the understanding that there might be something different about the cognitive self-awareness of an autistic person. Our hypothesis explains the developmental process specific to autism: autistic people have trouble constructing a sense of self because they can't process information quickly.

The belief that autism is an intellectual disability has lasted for a long time. Recent work in neuroscience has revealed new perspectives — for example, the work of Laurent Mottron and Michelle Dawson, who is herself autistic, at the University of Montreal in 2014. They argue that the autistic brain is wired in a way that prioritizes particular types of information, including visual information, which results in a form of intelligence that is merely *different*. Autistic intelligence appears to be more visual than verbal.

When sensory perception began to appear in official definitions of autism and in what autistic people were saying about their experiences, it was postulated that autism was a modulation or sensory processing disorder. Neuroscience is currently studying the "sensory reactivity" of autistic people, for which special autistic brain wiring is responsible. For example, in the early 2000s, the American neurologist Nancy Minshew set out her theory of connectivity and under-connectivity: autism is characterized by under-connectivity of high-level neural connections, but over-connectivity of local connections in the cortex.

Since 1985, following the example of Temple Grandin, several autistic adults have written about the particularities of the autistic brain, but this work has received little attention. However, autistic people the world over are saying the same thing, and what they say is supported by neuroscience. The common threads of autism are beginning to appear.

As we saw earlier, the research of Brigitte Chamak, who studies social representation theory in relation to autism, confirms that when autistic people talk about autism, they aren't talking about the same thing as people who are not affected. Whereas neurotypical people talk about communication, socialization, restricted interests, stereotyped behaviour, and even problems with sensory integration, autistic people evoke instead the particularities of perception and processing of information and emotions. Neurotypical people describe autism in terms of problems, in comparison with the way their own brains work, which they see as normal; autistic people describe autism simply as a particular way of functioning — their own way.

In summary, if we define autism as a particular way of functioning with certain common features, one that varies in intensity depending on the individual, and whose associated challenges are unique to each individual, we can gather the various theories and begin to understand the overall issue, an issue that is far more important and is likely to be physiological. Even if a comprehensive understanding of autism depends on brain research that has not yet been completed, the multi-perspective approach taken here will help us respond to the questions posed in this book.

Autism spectrum disorder (ASD) is recognized as a neurodevelopmental disorder: this statement will be our founding principle. The origins of ASD are still unknown, even if we strongly suspect that there is a genetic component. For the Canadian psychiatrist Peter Szatmari, ASD is the most complex of all neurodevelopmental disorders; according to Laurent Mottron, we are dealing with a brain structure whose ability to process information involves a genetic difference from that of the neurotypical brain.

We believe that autistic people have the same equipment as all humans, but that their brains are wired differently. The unusual connectivity of the autistic brain entails related differences in development and internal organization that oblige the body to move in certain ways. This is called autistic manifestation, and it occurs in the majority of autistic people the world over. It is often confused with behavioural problems, but it is not the same thing. These body movements have their own function: they represent the body's efforts to come to the brain's assistance when its particular wiring does not allow continuous and stable information processing. Rather than trying to suppress these behaviours and gestures in autistic people, we should allow them to happen in order to encourage the individual's development.

We are proposing that autism has two faces. We call these the hidden face — that of neural wiring — and the visible face — bodily movements. When the hidden side is in difficulty, it prompts the visible side to help. This is one reason some people have trouble understanding autism. The absence of a visible struggle means that they don't take the person's autistic functioning into account and, if the situation degenerates, they assume the person has a behavioural problem. Even professionals have been tricked by the visible face: if it disappears because the autistic manifestations are suppressed, they believe they have cured the autism! But the original problem lies with the neural connections, not the physical movements, and just because the wiring cannot be seen does not mean that it is not causing difficulties. Remember that autism is a neurodevelopmental disorder: it can evolve in a positive direction — the autistic person can learn to manage their autistic functioning — but it cannot be cured. It is not an illness from which people need to recover.

Most autistic people have no intellectual disability. We believe the confusion between autism and intellectual disability is a major problem, one that prevents us from realizing the rich human potential of autistic people. We believe it is crucial to intervene so as to respect the integrity of autistic people and give them quality of life.

Here are the premises of our position:

- We must understand how autism works.
- Lack of understanding of autistic functioning causes a great deal of anxiety in autistic people.
- We cannot ignore autistic functioning or make it disappear; it is part of the individual's identity and we must live with it.
- Autistic people speak a different language.
- It is possible to communicate with autistic people.
- Autism itself is not the cause of problems with behaviour or aggression; usually, an aggressive autistic individual is someone who has been the object of aggression.

As the field develops, we can see the conception of ASD evolving.

It's important to understand that no single approach is sufficient to describe autism. We believe that in order see the bigger picture, we must consider all aspects of autism — genetic, neurological, medical, developmental, behavioural, etc. Rather than opposing different practices, we should examine the results of experiments along with the corresponding metrics and hypotheses. The data advanced to promote a given theory are often highly selective and subjective because, in the majority of cases, the theory responds to the needs of neurotypical people. How can we confirm that a tool or a program meets the needs of autistic people when we are only just beginning to see certain points on the map of the autistic brain and to understand, among other things, the phenomenon of desynchronization of areas of the brain?

Although neurologists are in a position to see and measure dysfunction in the brain, only autistic people can bear witness to the physical and psychological effects of this particular brain wiring. It is only by combining advances in neuroscience with evidence from autistic people that we will be better able to understand their needs — and prove our hypothesis and the program that is associated with it.

2

What Is Autism?

AUTISM SPECTRUM DISORDER is a neurodevelopmental disorder. This means that the way the brain is connected (the particular wiring of the neural connections) has an impact on development. In fact, there are many studies that show anatomical difference in autistic brains. These anomalies change the brain's architecture. Specialists such as Rémy Lestienne are convinced that autism is due to "a deficiency or an anomaly in the pruning of neural synapses during embryonic life, and to the reorganization of neural connections at the end of adolescence." Studies in neuroscience show that the autistic brain is over-connected in certain localized areas and under-connected in areas that are farther apart, which may cause synchronization problems between these zones. This affects the overall "balance" of the brain, and when there is an imbalance, some normal developmental milestones cannot be reached.

> *Brigitte:* Autism isn't something we have, it's what we are. Your neurotypical brain isn't something you have, it's what you are. And since you aren't just that, neither are we!

This is a useful point at which to explain certain ideas that we will be referring to throughout this book. Some concepts and terms are also defined in the glossary at the end.

When we talk about balance, we mean the stable state that the whole organism tries to maintain in order to survive. This is homeostasis, a fundamental principle that characterizes not only the human body but every biological system. A perturbed system will try to keep its internal balance by reverting to its initial state — for example, if we are cold, the body adapts by generating more body heat. The brain can consciously decide that it is time to turn up the heat in the room. If we are very hot, our bodies will sweat in an attempt to cool down.

External information is constantly changing, as is our perception. Autistic people manage the link between the changing environment and their own bodies differently. Neurotypical people can adapt internally to a change in environment quickly and without visible effort. The neurotypical brain can react to a feeling of cold, for example, based on previous experience, because it can easily create reaction strategies from what it has previously learned. Autistic people also feel cold, but don't always know what to do with that fact because they are simultaneously besieged by other information. They must therefore "manually" or "consciously" handle the data their senses are reporting.

Their bodies try to respond to this information without the help of reaction strategies because their brains can't search for them. All their neural resources are being directed toward sensory input.

Think of a stable, balanced state as a balloon filled with little moving marbles. From time to time you might push the balloon gently to set the marbles into harmonious motion again (Figure 1A). Since the marbles' movement is constantly affected by external variations such as temperature and air currents (Figure 1B), you need to keep pushing the balloon gently to reposition the marbles and end up with a fluid movement (Figure 1C). This movement illustrates the efforts of internal rebalancing in the face of constantly changing external information. The ability to do this rebalancing work allows people to use their energy elsewhere, for example, in cognitive function.

We believe — and current research confirms — that the work of internal rebalancing can be learned because the plasticity of the brain, that is, its ability to modify connections in neural networks as a result of lived experiences. Treatments that help autistic people achieve the

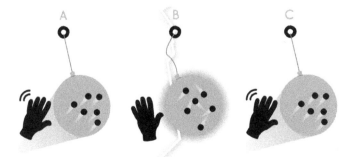

Figure 1: Homeostasis and the search for equilibrium

neural equilibrium they need to move on to new stages of development are ones that focus on plasticity and promote the creation of reaction strategies for different situations. Since mature brains retain their plasticity, even adults can attain these stages of development. Ultimately, this means that there is no age limit for seeking a better quality of life. It's important to understand that although autism remains present, it evolves, so there is always a way to improve an individual's functioning.

Neuroscience has shown that these wiring differences effectively mean that the autistic brain is wired in a "perceptive" way. The perceptive brain prioritizes concrete information — anything that is not social or based on details. This feature of the brain is independent of the individual's will. Autistic people notice the ceiling panels in a room rather than the people in that room. Their brains will tell them almost instantly how many ceiling panels there are, but will tell them nothing about the mood of the people.

CHARACTERISTICS OF THE AUTISTIC BRAIN

The brain wiring of people with ASD creates differences in sensory perception and language. First of all, autistic people have an increased sensitivity to the sensory environment. Studies increasingly show that this is a problem of over-connection: the perceptive brain takes in too much information and is unable to remove it from its thoughts. The brain must learn to adjust how much information is taken in to avoid sensory overloading.

This means that if an autistic individual jumps all the time, there's no need to put her on a trampoline so she can jump even more. The reason for the jumping has to do with balancing the relation between the body and its movement, not the sensations of the body or its position in space. Autistic people cannot move to the next stage of development by themselves; in helping them develop the cognitive mechanism that leads to the organization of thought, we help them to situate themselves in space and then to move. Some people need to touch the walls and furniture as they move around the edge of a room; others are always sitting on the floor. Their cognitive development means their movements will not be limited to the immediate environment.

Autistic people also have particular ways of processing information. We might compare the brain to a gearbox. Imagine that neurotypical people are equipped with an automatic transmission that takes care of all kinds of tasks smoothly behind the scenes, while autistic people have a manual transmission (Figure 2). In fact, they must consciously deal with every single scrap of information one piece at a time, with cognitive effort, which explains — among other things — their low processing speed. If you are autistic, everything comes in through the eyes, whether it be touch, image, or sound. The information that comes in must be dealt with one item at a time by a brain that only deals with things it recognizes and with which it can associate a reaction strategy. Obviously, managing a "manual" brain is a constant effort: many autistic people get exhausted easily and some have bad headaches for days on end. We must remember that even if autistic people don't say they are in pain, their bodies are hurting.

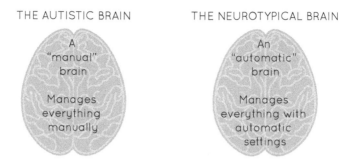

Figure 2: The manual brain and the automatic brain

Ultimately, the way the autistic brain develops means that autistic people need a language created for them, just as deaf people have sign language and blind people have Braille. At the SACCADE Centre D'Expertise en Autisme (Centre for Autism Expertise) in Quebec, we have developed a special language for autistic people — SACCADE Conceptual Language, or SCL — in order to allow them to communicate more easily, more usefully, and with improved organization of thought.

This is not about getting people to talk. An autistic person who cannot speak can be compared to a non-verbal deaf person: it's the deafness that's preventing speech, but teaching deaf people to speak will not "cure" their deafness. It's the same with autism: simply getting people to speak does not "solve" their autism. Besides, any speech obtained in this way comes from the perceptive side of the brain, not from the interactive side, the side where real communication develops. This is why most autistic people who have started to speak without going through a process of cognitive organization are stuck in echolalia, stereotyped language, or language with thematic repetition. The only thing they've learned is oral production.

BECOMING A SOCIAL BEING

The perceptive brain has trouble with several aspects of interaction: abstraction, reaction to a human voice, awareness of self and other, and social clues. Autistic people are "socially blind" from birth, to varying degrees. Some autistic people learn to decode concrete signs over time, but others never do. You can't teach someone to be "socially sighted"; it's more a matter of moving through a series of developmental stages. Development cannot be taught; it must be lived. Professionals who have, over the years, taught autistic people "socializing by rote" (eye contact, paying attention, social skills) have only added to what they learn by rote.

All human beings are programmed to become social creatures. To our knowledge, science has not yet demonstrated this is any different among autistic people, so we should continue to believe that they too are programmed to become social creatures. However, autistic people prioritize perception over socialization and communication, because their neural resources always address whatever is most urgent. Social information can indeed provoke an emotion in autistic people, but just like any other piece of data captured by the senses, this information has to go through the brain's cognitive organization to be processed. This mechanism will either provide the person with the meaning of the information or not: the information might remain devoid of meaning.

In a social situation, both brain and body will be required in maintaining internal equilibrium. Social interaction is possible once that equilibrium is reached. But if the social information that reaches the autistic person is too

> *Lise:* If a person sighs because they are tired from being with an autistic individual, that individual will not grasp the meaning of the action and will therefore be unable to use it to adjust their behaviour. He will probably be accused of being rude if he doesn't go away. But would we accuse a deaf person of being rude if she didn't answer someone who said hello, when she didn't hear or see them? *The autistic person cannot process what he does not see; the fact that his brain is wired differently means that his brain does not "see" social meaning.*

complex, the perceptive brain will not be able to process it while still trying to maintain equilibrium. The brain will therefore enlist its natural ally, the body. This is how the movements made by autistic people all over the world help the brain reconfigure itself in real time. The human body is intelligent: whether autistic or neurotypical, it uses everything it needs to maintain internal equilibrium. The body never does anything at random.

Autistic movements play a very important developmental role. The research does not indicate any benefit to making autistic people stop movements such as hand flapping. We believe that the purpose of such movements has been misunderstood because the map of how the autistic brain works has not yet been fully drawn and because we haven't taken into account the evidence of autistic people themselves. Nor do we know the consequences of forcibly stopping these movements, which is disturbing: no one has considered that. However, as soon as the brain can work alone, the movements stop by themselves. They may come back at times when processing information is more complicated (if the information itself is complex or if the person is tired or anxious). For the autistic person, complex information means information that has to be processed by the body coming to the brain's assistance, as well as by the brain itself.

THE THREE CHARACTERISTICS OF THE AUTISTIC BRAIN

We believe that all autistic people have three characteristics in common, regardless of the degree of severity or whether the autism is visible or not:

1. **Difficulty with brain initiative** — the brain always acts as though it needs an external push to set it in motion and move on to the next stage. Depending on the degree of severity, an autistic individual may not be able to create by herself the connections needed to move on to the next stage of development.

2. **Difficulty with abstraction**. Since their brains are visual and concrete, autistic people don't take in the invisible, including abstraction, inter-action, and socialization. The brain is wired to be perceptive rather than social, which makes autistic people "socially blind." Autistic people are reputed to be visual thinkers, but the reality is far more complex than that.

3. **Difficulty recalling information in real time**, or a delay in processing experiences, even in verbal

descriptions coming long after the event itself. The brain cannot process information relating to itself in real time. This is why we often hear autistic people replying "I don't know" in response to a personal question about their actual experience. This can be wrongly taken to mean that autistic people have no emotions.

In neurotypical brains, information coming from the outside world or the body is processed fluidly, almost automatically. For autistic people, each piece of information is processed as if it's a one-off: this is how autistic brains operate. A lack of equilibrium in autistic brain management provokes spectacular autistic crises (often inappropriately referred to as "meltdowns"). We have observed different degrees of crisis that seem to us to be difficulties with neural, cognitive, and psychological synchronization.

We believe that the severity of the autism corresponds to the gap between under- and over-connection, and to the lack of interaction between the senses, which requires manual processing of sensory information. The greater the gap between over- and under-connectivity, between non-social information that is easily processed and social information that can be processed only with great difficulty, the more severe the autism. This gap causes problems for both organizing thoughts and cognitive structure, making abstraction difficult. It also makes it harder to access emotions and to be aware of self and others; it slows down the retrieval of lived experience.

We believe that an approach that takes into account the neurodevelopmental side of autism will allow equilibrium and neuronal synchronization to be stabilized in such a way as to speed up cognitive organization, reduce the delay in processing information, and increase access to cognitive self-awareness, which is a fundamental stage. A brain that is in equilibrium and whose zones are working together is one that is able to develop.

CONCLUSION

Autism is a cerebral wiring problem whose effects are developmental. It involves particular strategies for dealing with information because the brain works differently. Autistic people interpret the world differently but are not cut off from the world; rather, they are cut off from the meaning of incoming information.

We need to see autism the same way we see deafness and blindness, because autistic people are "socially blind." They are deprived from birth of social clues because of the way their brains are wired: over-connected in some areas and under-connected in others, developing differently from neurotypical ones. This means, among other things, that emotional triggers are different, as is the way the person moves through the stages of emotional development. Autistic people don't deliberately behave a certain way, whether their autism is visible or not. Some autistic people face major difficulties, but for others the condition can also bring exceptional abilities.

Most autistic people are in survival mode. They are stuck between the real physical effects on their brain and the demands of the people around them. They can't ask for help, nor can they be helped by teaching, because the people around them lack the means to communicate with them. Autistic people are constantly forced back on their own resources. They may suffer enormously from this, yet still try to adapt to the world around them, just as neurotypical people do. For years we believed the opposite to be true, and this has had dreadful consequences for autistic people.

In the following chapters, we present questions that neurotypical people may ask, questions that arise from widespread misconceptions and to which we provide some answers. In this book we develop fifty or so ideas about autistic functioning and offer several pieces of advice that are based on a new understanding of ASD. This understanding is based on our theory of the internal function of autistic people, and is starting to resonate more and more widely among health and education professionals.

3

Manifestations of Autism

1.   Why Is He Always Off In His Own Little World?

➤   **Myth: Autistic people live in a world of their own.**

This is one of the biggest, oldest myths we need to destroy.

People talk a great deal about "being in their own world" in relation to autistic people. Even though this is a common expression, its meaning is misunderstood, because it doesn't mean what you might expect. People use this term because autistic people appear to be alone with themselves; they seem not to pay attention to the people around them, or don't reply when they are spoken to. This is when they are said to be "in their own little world."

We can compare this to a computer in sleep mode, or even to someone with their head in the clouds. When they're in their own world, autistic people are conscious but information doesn't quite reach them. It's as if information were trapped behind a pane of glass, or someone were speaking on the other side of a window.

It does not mean that the person is in an emotional bubble: autism is not an emotional disorder but a perceptive one. So being in one's own world also has to do with perception; it is directly related to information processing. In their own world, the autistic person cannot organize thoughts, can't speak, and remains static. It's as if the nervous system that captures information from both the outside world and inside the body has broken down. The different zones of the brain do not seem to be communicating, almost as if they were sulking. When we refer to remediation, we're talking about the work necessary to improve neuronal synchronization so that the different zones of the brain can communicate with one another.

The autistic "world" is not impermeable. Autistic people live in the same world as everyone else, but their static brains have a unique way of functioning, and they process incoming information differently.

> We can explain the "off in their own world" effect today through the internal workings of the autistic brain. There is work to be done to help autistic people progress to the next stage of development.

2. Why Is He Banging His Head?

We hear things like "She's self-harming" when an autistic person bangs her head. We need to distinguish between autistic manifestations and behavioural problems. People who make this kind of comment are simply showing their ignorance of the issue.

When the incoming information is too complex to handle, the autistic brain experiences a destabilization like an internal earthquake or storm. This storm has a physical manifestation. The reflex of the autistic person is to try to recover stability, often by trying to put pressure on a particular area in the upper part of the head. This region is very sensitive in autistic people because it corresponds to the position of the "centre console" of the manual brain that allows the autistic person to control themselves. It isn't uncommon to see autistic people hit themselves on the head if nobody goes to help them. They have no intention of self-harming or self-stimulating; rather, it's a survival mechanism provoked by a very uncomfortable physical phenomenon, accompanied by enormous unease. In such circumstances, the person needs help.

This "survival" mechanism starts off a chain reaction that gives access to the work of cognitive organization, which leads to self-awareness. It's crucial for an autistic person to learn to control this mechanism as soon as it becomes present and accessible.

People have long believed that the appearance of this survival mechanism indicates behavioural problems, instead of being a physical reaction to stimuli, something like when we feel the need to scratch. However, the autistic person needs help, and there are interventions and techniques that can be taught to help calm the internal earthquake and facilitate self-regulation.

3. Why Do Autistic Children Never Stop Moving?

Why is my child always moving around and unable to concentrate on one activity for long? He moves around the room constantly, flitting from one thing to another; sometimes he stops to watch cars passing in the street, but he soon starts moving again.

Unlike neurotypical people, autistic individuals are managing the relationship between external information and their body's internal state all the time. If the brain perceives an external change, their internal equilibrium is disturbed and the person must re-establish this equilibrium accordingly. He is moving to try to find or return to a state of equilibrium. For him, movement is his body's normal physical reaction to the demands made on his brain by changes he perceives in his environment.

Since everything external is changing all the time, autistic people prioritize the search for internal equilibrium, which takes place through constant movement. The human body does not move at random; this is a survival mechanism.

> The work that needs to be done on the autistic brain —
> that is, creating reaction strategies for different external
> stimuli — will reduce the individual's need to move, so she
> can focus her resources elsewhere, for example on cognitive function.

Kim: Since we used to see Valmond constantly moving, we thought he needed physical activity. We took him skiing, sledding, skating, cycling, swimming, and even to Sky Venture, where he literally flew, the way parachutists do during freefall. Valmond even had a season pass to the La Ronde amusement park, where he could go back to the same ride nine times in a row. But for the last few years, Valmond has refused to go on his favourite rides, which are the ones where you get dizziest. Over the past year, he's become thoughtful, too. He watches us from his chair, hardly moving. His father even wondered if Valmond was becoming depressed. But you only have to look at his face to see that he's interested in the world around him, and that he can follow what's going on without moving. He can concentrate on colouring for 30, 45, or even 60 minutes without a break, and at school he can sit and complete a piece of work without interruption. He will now stop swimming or sledding when he's had enough. Valmond still flits from one thing to another in a chaotic or new situation, of course. But in general, he has become more zen than I am.

4. Why Don't Autistic People Want Me to Touch Them?

➤ **Myth: Autistic people don't like being touched.**

The scientific literature confirms that autistic people of all ages don't like being touched. At the beginning of their journey with a child on the autism spectrum, some parents notice that they can't hug their child or caress his skin without making him extremely uncomfortable. This is hard for a parent to understand and cope with.

Brigitte: I always wear clothes with long sleeves when I'm around people, to avoid collecting marks from people around me. If I don't see a person's touch — if I can't associate the physical sensation of the touch with seeing a person putting a hand on my shoulder — I'm likely to "carry" that mark around with me for hours. The mark works its way into my skin and stays there. It's very uncomfortable, and sometimes exhausting and painful.

Kim: Like all parents do, I used to wait on the sidewalk for Valmond to come home from school. When he got off the bus, I would rush toward him, touching him and bombarding him with questions: "How are you?" "Are you tired?" "Mommy's made you some fish" … Ten times out of ten, Valmond avoided me and ran quickly into the house. For the next little while he would hide out on the sofa, his fingers stuck in his ears, sweating like crazy.

After Brigitte and Lise explained to me that I was causing Valmond discomfort by being in his face, I started remaining seated until he was ready. He would then come to me, moving my hair so he could smell my neck before kissing me on my eyelids, my cheeks, my head, and under my chin. I stayed still and quiet so he could see me. I stayed still and quiet so as not to rush him. I stayed still and quiet to love him at his pace, in his way. It's actually quite logical: you can't love a fish by petting it like a dog. Valmond managed to completely change my behaviour.

It is well known that autistic people prefer long clothes that prevent them from getting "stuck" if they touch someone's skin or an unknown texture. Unseen touch sparks discomfort and leaves a disagreeable "mark" behind. This mark lingers until the brain can process the related sensory information.

For autistic people, touch is very complex. Everything comes in through the eyes: if a touch isn't seen, or if the brain can't associate an image with the physical sensation being felt, it can't be registered, so it actually causes genuine discomfort. This isn't emotional discomfort; autistic people are actually facing the conceptual problems associated with information processing. Physical contact has to be seen for the message to be relayed to the brain.

As soon as they sense contact, autistic people's brains start processing the incoming sensory information. Until this information has been processed and categorized, the brain cannot process anything new. Neurotypical people might have a similar reaction when they are wearing clothing with a label that irritates the skin on their neck or back. It is difficult to concentrate on the present moment until the label issue is sorted out. Once the label is out of the way, the person will be ready to move on to something else immediately, whereas autistic people will live with the feeling of the label for hours to come.

This phenomenon, which is caused by the autistic brain's over-connectivity, should not be confused with the problem of sensory processing. Nor is it an emotional issue. Whether the contact comes from a person or an unknown texture, the perceptive over-connectivity of the autistic brain acts as if this is "too much," and puts it in the queue of information to be processed. This way of processing information is the same for all incoming stimuli: tactile, auditory, and visual.

> When you touch an autistic person for the first time, or when the person is in a new situation or is feeling tired or anxious, you should never move, or speak, or ask them anything. You should simply touch in a static way: without moving, letting your hand remain still. In this way you will help the autistic person to speed up how they process this touch; afterwards, when they are used to this static touching, you can gradually introduce non-static touching. The autistic person will ultimately be able to process this contact more easily.

5. Why Do Autistic People Object to the Sounds of Lawnmowers, Hairdryers, and Other Tools and Appliances? Is It Normal to Wear Earphones All Day?

The sounds of many electrical appliances and tools, such as drills, lawnmowers, coffee grinders, hairdryers, and smoke alarms, can upset autistic people. The noise triggers a reaction that can look disproportionate, but it shows the person's genuine fear and pain.

These noises are like environmental assaults on the over-connected autistic brain. Autistic people seem to have heightened reactions to environmental sensory stimuli.

Lise: Because autistic people are overloaded with information from different external stimuli, they tire very quickly. They need a calm environment for work and rest. We always need to make sure they are rested before taking them to busy places like malls, and that they are receptive enough to manage the noise, the new people, and the various stimuli of public places. When an outing doesn't go well, we should determine whether they are tired out from too much stimulation.

The sound of a coffee maker might seem wavelike: it's not regular, but uneven and unpredictable, full of little variations that the autistic person can't quite grasp. It's not the noise but its irregular quality that assaults the information-processing system.

Autistic people can quickly be exhausted by such noises and will instinctively try to avoid them. These noises "hurt" them; in other words, they cause an actual physical pain inside the head, but one that's nothing like, for example, the pain of stubbing your toe. An irregular noise is an aggression that keeps resonating, continuing until it can be processed. In this way autistic people show a kind of sensory acuity, a sensitivity that is out of their control.

The sound of a lawnmower can be "seen": in order to identify and process it, autistic people must be able to associate the noise with the tool producing it, at the time that it's producing it. The lawnmower must be fixed in time and space, otherwise there will be unease: will this thing make a noise for the rest of my life? But be careful: if all you do is show the autistic person the lawnmower and show it

Brigitte: I avoid changing the batteries in my alarm system because the noise is very harsh. Irregular noises like those of alarm systems can cause enormous pain inside my head, in a precise spot far from my ears. It's not my ears that hurt, but the part of my head where I visually associate sound information with its source. Because I need to see the noise, its irregularity is a problem for me: it's too much different information to process at the same time. Mission impossible!

Noise is even more difficult to decode when someone is speaking. The problem is that there's no synchronization between the noise coming in from one side and the voice coming from the other, even though my eyes are trying to match images to everything coming in through my ears. So I have to look at the speaker's mouth. It's easier that way.

It's the same phenomenon as touch or unstable images, yet fans and spinning tops don't cause me any problems.

Managing a manual brain is hard work.

stopping, it will forever be associated with that very precise sequence and will stay stuck in the same context, which will always have the same start and end point.

On the other hand, it's not normal to have to wear headphones all day long. That's actually a clue that the work of conceptualization hasn't been done. Doing this work is vital so that the autistic person can grasp the meaning of the information coming in.

It's true that autistic people are visual, but we must help them so that their minds make the necessary links. Their internal visual sense must be triggered to allow them to do the work of cognitive organization, otherwise all the links will be made by their external visual sense — the one that takes in the environment, not the one that organizes thought. In this way we take away the camera and offer them a video recorder that captures movement.

6. Why Do Autistic People Constantly Move Their Arms, Hands, and Heads? Is It Normal to Make Movements Like That?

In the literature, we speak of autistic manifestations. Often, when we see an autistic person flapping their arms like wings, waggling their fingers near their eyes, rocking, going up and down on tiptoe, or making other, similar movements, we try to make them stop, reasoning that these movements are not socially acceptable. As soon as the autistic person stops doing these things, everyone will think they've done their job. But why have we decreed that autistic people should not be allowed to express themselves by moving their bodies?

Back when we thought autism was an illness, autistic manifestations were considered symptoms to be eradicated. Nobody wondered why autistic people the world over made the same movements, nor what purpose they

> If we had wanted blind people to go around without being noticed, we wouldn't have made their canes white. It's the same with autistic people and their movements.
>
> — Laurent Mottron

served. However, to this day, no study has been able to show why they should be suppressed. Now that we know autism is a neurodevelopmental issue, autistic movements take on a different meaning. And we still don't know how forcing people to stop making these movements affects development.

When the brain struggles to process a complex piece of information, the whole body is enlisted to help it maintain a necessary equilibrium. We can describe the physical movements as signs of the body coming to the brain's assistance, and they fade away or disappear by themselves when the brain is able to manage the task alone.

Remember that the human body is intelligent and does nothing randomly. We should never try to stop autistic people from making these spontaneous movements. They are part of a developmental stage through which autistic people pass. The movements happen at a particular moment, and their presence tells us what intervention and support are appropriate. It's essential to keep in mind at all times the internal functioning and overall autistic wiring of the individual.

> Brigitte: It's not me making these movements — it's my body.

7. What Does Hand Flapping Mean?

Some people believe that they should prevent autistic people from hand flapping — a rapid hand movement common among autistic people. As soon as they have done it, they proclaim victory: the autism is "cured" because it is no longer visible! This is wrong. Hand flapping is not restricted to autistic people; it's actually typical of human development. All children around the age of nine months make this movement, and it disappears over time. Would we consider stopping a nine-month-old from moving their arms? Absolutely not! We would find beauty in a child expressing himself, and we would allow him to develop over time.

In autistic people, hand flapping shows up later and remains for longer. Many autistic people confirm this. We see it in two circumstances: as an indicator that the person is experiencing a positive emotion, or when there is a mix of emotions coming together before a crisis. The presence of hand flapping in autistic people is actually a welcome sign, because it indicates that a certain developmental stage has been reached. Hand flapping is the motor expression of an emotion, not a behaviour to be suppressed. It's a sign that the brain has become able to register positive emotions (for example, the person doing it is expressing contentment).

Hand flapping can be seen as a way the body helps the brain take in positive emotion — joy, an emotion that promotes communication. As soon as the brain has processed the information contained in this emotion, the hand flapping is no longer necessary; it becomes pointless and disappears by itself. We still don't know the effects on development of suppressing hand flapping. If we intervene at this stage, we must be very careful.

Since hand flapping is associated with a developmental stage related to emotions, we should celebrate its arrival, and then support the person in moving to the next stage. In some autistic people, hand flapping might remain throughout life, or reappear from time to time; this is not a negative thing, since it is still the motor expression of an emotion.

8. Why Are Autistic People Always Clutching Something in Their Hands? Why Do They Refuse to Let Go of These Objects?

Autistic people often carry objects in their hands: a small car or truck, a soft toy, a book, a paper clip, a ball, a pencil, a little radio, a Tangle. When someone tries to take them away, they react strongly.

An object held in the hand is wrongly seen as a transition object. For autistic people, it's actually something stable that helps them to situate their own body as they move through space. Whereas the position of the body is changing at every moment, requiring the autistic brain to keep seeking equilibrium, the object is concrete and stays constant. Its presence anchors the person in their physical reality and allows their cognitive functions to be deployed elsewhere.

When an autistic person starts to situate her physical presence in her environment, she touches the walls as if blind, which allows the brain to follow the body's movements, to locate itself in space. At a later stage, she will

Brigitte: My Tangle, a small object twisted in a certain way and designed to be held in the hand, is good for sending stable information to my brain about where my body is in a room. It helps me do an update and move on to other things. That way I don't need to touch the furniture or walls to size up my environment. My brain needs stable points of reference that don't change but can be moved. With a Tangle in my hand, I can move around without my brain needing to stop everything to concentrate on my movements. I have access to my thoughts without having to stop in order to think. This allows me spend my energy differently — on organizing my sentences or planning my movements.

use an object that she holds and that allows her to travel through an environment. The objects serves as a concrete measure for the brain, and the individual will be able to follow the body's movement in an environment and reach a higher level of decoding.

There's no particular age at which an autistic person uses a management object (such as a fidget toy or a tactile object). If you try to take an object of this kind away, the individual will react strongly — they are afraid of no longer being able to move around, because their brain will stop cooperating. They will need to go back to the known environment, touching the walls and furniture with their fingers, before being able to carry on the movement that was interrupted — or they will have trouble orienting themselves as they move.

> If an autistic person has to put down their management object for a moment, it's crucial to let them choose where they put it. They will probably leave it in sight so they can use it if they need it. Otherwise, they might become distressed.

9. People Say That Autistic People Are Inflexible and Their Brains Are Static. What's the Difference Between Inflexible and Static?

People point out that autistic people don't want things to change or be moved, and that they leave everything in the same place, always eat the same food and wear the same shoes. If not, there's a crisis!

When we say that autistic people are "inflexible," we are describing them inaccurately. They are not choosing to be intransigent, but are actually sending the message that their brains refuse to change certain images that they have saved and continue to carry. They need help. It's important to properly distinguish between the terms "static" and "inflexible."

An inflexible person demonstrates great rigidity: he follows rules to the letter and is unable to adapt. However, he can be dynamic in his information processing. His rigidity stems from how he deals with people and his environment; it is an external problem.

Being static means existing without changing, without moving, and without dynamism. Dynamic is the opposite of static. The autistic brain is static, not rigid. It's jerky and twitchy — it can't grasp continuous movement or process the

Brigitte: My brain receives information in sequential order and refuses to change it. I used to make my hot chocolate the following way: I got out my cup, put in the chocolate powder, and then poured in the water. This sequence was called "hot chocolate." One day, someone I'd invited to my house started to make me hot chocolate for a treat. She took my cup, poured in the water, and then added the powder. When I saw her do that, my brain started skipping as if an image I could see on Skype was freezing. I knew that it was possible to reverse the steps, but because my eyes took in the situation, my reaction was intense. It took a lot of energy for me to rebalance to "stabilize" my head.

Before I knew I was autistic, that kind of situation used to terrify me because it always took me by surprise. Now I know how my head works, I can predict such situations.

flow of information smoothly. This is an internal problem that has nothing to do with voluntary behavioural rigidity.

Imagine that autistic people have to supply a river with water, using a bucket to maintain the flow: it's irregular and exhausting work. While the brain is processing information, autistic people can experience an effect like a CD skipping, or a download freezing. The images become static without warning. That is what happens with a manual brain.

Using SACCADE Conceptual Language, or SCL, allows autistic people to find equilibrium in their bodies. After that, real cognitive organization follows; this will allow them to process information in ways that are more fluid and less static.

10. Why Do Autistic People Line Up Objects?

We have long observed that autistic people neatly line up all kinds of things. Small cars, pencils, toy alphabet letters, books, DVD cases … As soon as someone tries to tidy up, take out one of the things, or move what they've done, there's a catastrophe, and nobody knows why. What could the purpose of this behaviour be?

Lining up objects is perceived as a stereotypical behaviour that a parent or caregiver might try to stop without understanding its function. But why would many autistic people, no matter where they live on the planet, exhibit the same behaviour and the same movements, unless they had a particular purpose?

Kim: We're probably the only people who still have VHS tapes! Over the years we must have acquired around fifty; Valmond used to watch them when he was younger. For a couple of years now he's been lining them up on the ground and the table, like bricks rather than train carriages, with the tapes touching each other and following a precise order. And their distance from other objects in the room — the table, the rug — seems to be calculated to the centimetre.

From time to time, Valmond will deliberately replace one tape with another. He used to get very irritated and disrupted in his head when we had to move the tapes to sweep. But for the last year he's just replaced them without showing any annoyance. Basically, we have a permanent "art installation" in our living room, which has mostly become Valmond's living room.

Neurotypical information
processing: fluid

Autistic information
processing: jerky

Figure 3: The way neurotypical and autistic brains process information

We believe that this behaviour is associated with autistic brain wiring. It could be a sign that the person is exercising control by making a continuous sequence in the environment. She has moved beyond the stage of seeing everything consciously as individual snapshots, from one moment to the next, to a stage where all the snapshots are linked and form a sequence with a beginning and an end (Figure 3). This is how autistic people make sense of their environment. The ability to capture continuous movement is progress for them. We don't know the consequences of trying forcibly to stop this behaviour. Since the research has not distinguished between behaviours that might be essential for autistic development and harmful behaviours that should be prevented, we believe that putting small objects in rows is a stage in the autistic individual's development and we try to support this individual as they move toward a higher stage.

Brigitte: It's not so much the light that assaults autistic people as its irregular flickering.

11. Why Do Autistic People Like to Watch Fans and Tops Spinning?

Autistic people often like watching fans. They sit in front of them and calmly watch them spinning for several minutes.

The autistic brain processes what it recognizes. Watching tops spinning or fans turning stimulates information processing in autistic people because it's a stable, regular movement — known and predictable. The regularity of this movement gives autistic people a lot of pleasure.

When autistic individuals have reached certain stages of development, their information-processing system becomes more sophisticated and their comfort with this type of regularity will be transferred onto more complex tasks such as mathematics, calendars, public transit timetables, physics, and so on (Mottron 2004). Studying these regular systems has a calming effect on autistic people.

> It's not harmful to let the child watch an object spinning, as long as it's not for hours at a time. Remember that this corresponds to a developmental stage, and the child needs help to move on.

Conversely, any "unstable" or irregular stimulation, whether that's a noise, a light, or a touch, can make autistic people extremely uncomfortable. For example, fluorescent light produces a mixed spectrum of light rather than a continuous spectrum. Because that twisting light is a constant input for an over-connected brain, an autistic person can become exhausted without knowing why. It's important to avoid this type of lighting.

4

Daily Life

12. Why Is Getting a Haircut Such a Drama?

Parents often report that haircuts are very difficult for the autistic child. The child refuses, reacts strongly, cries, and expresses real fear. Parents have to come up with all kinds of strategies to achieve their goal — strategies that are often very anxiety-inducing for the child. Some parents sneak in a haircut while the child is asleep. Others choose to wait.

We now know that if a certain developmental stage has not been reached, autistic people don't know that hair grows back. They might believe that a haircut is for life! In addition, they have no real concept of time. Touching their hair means touching their "image," modifying an image that must remain stable for them. They can't make the image evolve in time because it's stuck in the present. Changing it by having a haircut therefore becomes very anxiety-inducing.

If the individual knows that hair grows, he doesn't necessarily know at what length, or when it should be cut. And if the length varies, that's even more confusing. His brain requires a stable reference to make sense of the experience, but it doesn't have one. If the idea that hair regrows is not internalized, the idea of cutting the hair is even less so.

In addition, noises "enter through the eyes." The noise of the clippers, which is unstable and irregular, might terrify a child if he can't make sense of it.

Lise: We succeeded one day in using visual tools to explain to four-year-old Xavier that his hair grew, that it needed to be cut, and that it would grow back again. We showed him the steps involved in a haircut. He then calmly accepted having his hair cut. Some hours later, while he was playing in his room, he stopped and put his hand on his head. We heard him say, "Oh no! It hasn't grown back yet!" He had understood the meaning of "cutting hair."

Kim: It took two of us to hold Valmond down so he could have his hair cut. Every time it was an enormous struggle, with Valmond screaming and us using the clippers for speed — as well as to shave it as short as possible to delay the next haircut.

Today, Valmond asks me to cut his hair every evening in the bath. I restrict myself to ten or fifteen snips of the scissors, but I can do as many as necessary. Valmond even shows me which bits to cut, because while he brushes his hair he is looking at — and recognizing — himself in the mirror. Once or twice he's even cut a rebellious strand himself.

Brigitte: I've never had a different haircut, because the image I have of myself is very static and must stay that way. Fashion has no effect on me: I don't understand why someone would want their hair short, then long, then red or blue! I hate it when other people change their hairstyle because I have trouble recognizing them. And I didn't go to the hairdresser until quite late in life. I still find hair salons difficult: everyone's talking; there's a lot of noise, lights, and smells; and the hairdresser has to keep touching my head as she works. That's a lot going on all at the same time!

13. Why Are Autistic People Afraid of Showers?

Parents report that their child refuses to take showers. They keep having to remind the child and insist on the shower, which is exhausting.

For autistic people, everything enters through the eyes. This includes touch. Every touch must be recorded by the eyes, even the sensation of water hitting skin. At a certain stage of noticing movement, the brain becomes a submachine gun as it marks each drop that touches the skin. An autistic person might be afraid of showers, or might simply say that the water "hurts" them.

At a different stage it's possible that, having no concept of time, an autistic person will not manage to deduce that a shower starts and ends. The individual won't be able cognitively to organize the events of the shower as they unfold. To complicate the matter further, trying to communicate to the child the idea of "the length of the shower" verbally

Brigitte: For autistic people, the idea of a "shower" is very complex. First, there's the physical environment: I have to move within this small space while I'm figuring out the environment. I can't change the shower curtain too often, because I need at all times to have the visual measure of my body in relation to its surroundings, one thing at a time. If the shower curtain changes, everything needs to be reconfigured! If I can't manage to decode the space, my brain refuses to follow.

Next, I have to process each drop of water falling on my skin as a separate piece of information. At the beginning, I used to see them one by one. It was hard work! Today, water's fine. I no longer feel the drops individually because my system is more functional; I can think of them abstractly, get in the shower, and plan to wash.

So, not only do I have to visually plan my movements inside the shower area, I also have to manage the irregular arrival of drops of water, plan to wash, correctly calculate the movements of the cloth, the effect of the soap, and the rinsing. There's a whole sequence of actions that must each be thought about "intentionally."

This is why having a shower is so complicated. But with patience and persistence, you can get there!

(for example, saying several times that it won't be long, just a few more minutes) is likely to fix that activity in time and make it "static."

An autistic child also doesn't know how to position his body in relation to the physical space of the shower (the floor, the walls, the ceiling), which makes the steps involved in washing the body very laborious. The unstable points of reference make him feel as if he's in a void every time. Every movement needed to wash part of his body demands a lot of concentration and energy.

Because their brains are over-connected, autistic people are aware of "every" drop of water on their skin. The brain can't process this, because it keeps being asked to process the other drops that keep landing. The first drop is followed by the second, which also demands to be processed once it touches the skin, so the eyes are immediately called on to process it.

> In the beginning, it's often easier to choose a bath instead of a shower. Otherwise, washing can become an anxiety-inducing activity, using up a lot of energy for no reason.

14. Is Autism the Reason My Seven-Year-Old Is Still Wearing Diapers?

Autism prevents some children from fully understanding toilet training at the same stage of development as neurotypical children.

Two different types of toilet training have to happen — urine and stools. As long as an autistic child hasn't understood the meaning of the activity, he won't be able to do it. Just as the meaning of other things enters through the eyes, the child needs to *see* what people are trying to teach.

There is no reason why an autistic child should not become toilet trained as long as there are no other disorders. On the other hand, toilet training might need to start a little later than it does for neurotypical people.

The strategies we often use in teaching children, such as reinforcement (rewards), mimicking peers, verbal instruction, and the desire to please adults, don't usually work for autistic children. It's pointless to try to toilet train an autistic child with a standard development timeline. Autistic children need to reach a certain maturity level, have a knowledge of their body in space, and visually understand what is being asked of them. Autistic children will need help with toilet training. Get out paper and pencil to explain it to them. And keep quiet when they're on the toilet trying to concentrate.

15. Why Is My Child Extremely Picky About Food, and Why Must Different Foods on His Plate Not Touch?

➤ **Myth: It's normal for autistic people not to eat much. Autistic people are very inflexible when it comes to food.**

This is not true. Eating is very complex for autistic people. It's a conceptual problem rather than a sensory one, caused by the brain's static quality and its fixed images. The effect of the autistic brain is significant here. It might be that an autistic person, at a certain developmental stage, doesn't recognize hunger, and the references he has for understanding that he needs to eat are all external. For example, the individual might want to eat only from his blue plate, otherwise it's not a meal. She might only want to eat Mom's spaghetti, because Grandma's isn't the same at all, even if it's made from the same recipe. He might want to drink water only from his yellow cup, and refuse anything else. She might restrict her menu to just five foods and not get bored with them. Food that's warmer or colder than usual might go uneaten.

If the people around the autistic individual don't understand, and if the references are all external and environmental, meals will become increasingly trying moments.

The conceptual overload of mealtimes causes many problems for autistic people, particularly the inconsistent nature of the texture and shape of the food. At a certain stage of development, an autistic person cannot understand the meaning of food. She might not know that the object she is being given on her usual plate is in fact food, simply because its shape is different. Carrots served as coins are not the same thing as carrots cut into sticks. The image is completely different, as is the internal reference.

An autistic person might also be focusing his brain on eating, and directing his mental resources there. If people around him are interacting, it might prevent him from concentrating on eating. For this reason, many autistic people refuse to eat or sit down with other people at the table. Some will tell us to be quiet because they are eating.

Because the autistic person doesn't identify hunger, think of eating, or consider meals as having a social function, some autistic people can't understand why we sit down, or why we have to eat the food given to us. For many, mealtimes are not social activities, but rather an obligatory task — eating in order to stay healthy.

Brigitte: Food and meals have always been very difficult for me. I spent years looking at pictures or reading while I ate because I couldn't look at the people around me. I needed to avoid exposing myself to visual stimuli during the meal so I could concentrate on the act of eating. Hearing people talk around me was just as disturbing.

I also have a lot of trouble with textures. When a food is reheated, it's not the same anymore. If a single ingredient in a recipe is changed, it's no longer the same recipe. Everything I eat must be known and recognized. This was a big problem for several years. I could only eat a few foods. And I drowned everything else in ketchup!

The different kinds of food couldn't touch one another on my plate, otherwise they would lose their visual coherence and I would no longer recognize the image I was seeing. It was the same with my glass of milk: if the amount was different, it was no longer a glass of milk.

Meals were often complicated. Today, I vary my food a little more, but I still have trouble with texture and with food changing identity!

If the autistic person must still capture the meaning of information visually, nothing will tell him that the time to leave the table is when dessert is over. Because the kind and quantity of food are never the same, it can be difficult to figure out when to get up from the table. So to understand what's going on, some people always ask for the same foods, others ask for food that is the same colour, still others ask for exactly the same amount, and so on.

Kim: My son would only ever eat the soft part of crois-sants. One day, my mother turned the croissant inside out, hiding the crust on the inside. Valmond took the mouthful without hesitating. From this, we concluded that it was the visual aspect rather than the texture that bothered him. Valmond would separate the ham-burger from its bun, chicken from rice, sausage from pasta … Another time, my mother pushed some meat inside a ball of rice to trick Valmond. He spat it out every time, which showed us that it was the mixture of tastes, or perhaps the texture, that he was rejecting. Because Valmond is non-verbal, we spend a lot of time trying to guess what he finds upsetting, agreeable, irri-tating, off-putting … comforting. Today, if we reintro-duce one ingredient at a time, at his pace, Valmond can suggest his own mixtures of flavours by putting every-thing he wants in one meal on the table. These days we can ask him if he would prefer pasta or potatoes, a bagel or a tortilla …

However, he is still a mystery. We will never know why he gave up ketchup overnight — something that he added to every meal for the first five years of his life. One day, he suddenly rejected it, to the point of refusing to allow a bottle in our grocery cart. My late father-in-law would have been happy, since he believed that the sauce altered the taste of food. Perhaps Valmond had been trying to make the taste of his meals uniform by drowning them in ketchup.

It's pointless to insist at all costs that an autistic person eat everything that's put in front of them until the work of cognitive organization is done. Autistic people need to eat to survive. This isn't a sensory issue, as has long been thought, but rather a conceptual task. It is strongly recommended not to do this work during mealtimes, but rather as a separate activity.

It's preferable to reduce the number of potential environmental stimuli (television, music, noise, etc.), so that an autistic person can eat her meal. Calm is helpful. There is no point trying to work on several major areas of learning at the same time. You need to choose the individual's priorities.

Children three and older can be shown the meaning of meals with the book *Tedou mange.**

16. Why Do Autistic People React So Strongly to a Little Scratch on Their Arm, but Not at All to a Fractured Femur?

➤ **Myth: Autistic people don't feel pain.**

Parents tell us this all the time: their child falls down the stairs and breaks a bone without showing any signs of pain. But getting a simple scratch on the finger is a major trauma.

Information goes in through the eyes. Autistic people see the scratch, outside themselves, and see that it changes

---

* The Tedou series, written by Brigitte Harrisson and Lise St-Charles, was created specifically for autistic children.

Brigitte: I've had a few worrying experiences because I struggled to locate pain. One day at work, I had stomach ache for an hour or so around lunchtime. Afterwards, things went back to normal and I finished up my workday. I drove an hour to get home. That evening, when I wanted to eat, the pain came back. A friend advised me to see a doctor. The following day, I had an urgent operation. When I woke up, I was missing my appendix, one ovary, and my uterus! I had had appendicitis, and since I also have endometriosis, an enormous ovarian cyst had burst. I was being poisoned from the inside and the surgeons had to clean everything up. I hadn't noticed any sign of it, except for a stomach ache that lasted between 30 and 60 minutes and whose intensity hadn't really worried me.

the configuration of their skin, but they do not see the break, which is inside their body. The brain therefore cannot grasp this information and see it as a priority.

The scratch changes the person's image of their body, which is enough to make the autistic person doubt the version they had of it. A child with a scratched finger can no longer function; she is obsessed with her "new" finger, by the new image of her body that she has to make. She isn't crying because of the pain of the scratch, but because she is afraid of the change that has just happened. She doesn't know that her skin isn't ruined forever. Since she has no concept of time, she can't move her self-image in time and update it with this modified version.

However, even though the information processing doesn't render the pain conscious, the injured body is indeed in pain. We must not neglect the physical health of an autistic person, because a body that somatizes (turns psychological discomfort into physical pain) still experiences a pain that is perceived as distant, like background noise. If an autistic person breaks their leg, they will limp, and they might even be irritable without knowing why. At this stage of development, even if they are verbal, they can't express their pain verbally.

> If an autistic person does not do the necessary brain development work, he will remain seemingly insensitive to pain.

17. When Autistic People Go Out of the House in Winter, Why Don't They Cover Up, and Why Don't They Feel Cold?

People who spend time with autistic individuals often say how hard it is to get them to wear warm clothes outside, because they never show that they are cold, and it is up to the person in charge to make sure that they are not in danger. Autistic people of any age can get frostbite without realizing it.

Why? Because cold cannot be seen! To grasp a sensation, an autistic individual has to find it visually, with their eyes, and compare it to a known reference ("it's hot" in relation to "it's cold"). As long as everything has to be identified by the eyes, the body won't respond on its own.

Unlike neurotypical people, autistic individuals cannot automatically respond to the feeling of being cold,

Kim: When he was little, Valmond refused to wear his snowsuit. Once, we took him out without dressing him for a few seconds so that he could understand the cold. Unfortunately, we soon realized that Valmond had not made the link between the cold and the purpose of winter clothes. For years, we used to have to run after him to wrap him up. If we didn't, he would go out in −20°C in a T-shirt without understanding why his body was shivering. Once he began to associate the discomfort of cold with the solution to the discomfort of cold, he started coming back to put on not only his coat but also his hat and gloves. Also, when he came back with cold feet, he slipped them under my legs and put his hands on my neck. In the same way, he became capable of expressing a pain that wasn't visible: saying "booboo" while showing me the foot that he'd hit on a corner of the table, spontaneously letting out an "ouch," or asking me to take care of him by saying "cream."

because their brains cannot interpret the sensation according to previous experience and give an order to solve the problem. The brain perceives cold, but it doesn't always know what to do with that information, because it is also besieged by other sensations to which the body is trying to respond. It can't use reaction strategies that it hasn't learned. Even if it has already learned them, it doesn't always use them, because its resources are focusing on perception. When the autistic person has created reaction strategies for different stimuli and is able to conceptualize cold, she will be able to interpret the temperature and react appropriately.

Brigitte: I never really used to feel cold outside, nor heat. I had boiling hot baths. I used to turn red all over, like a lobster! I used to read for hours in the bath, and as soon as the water started to cool down, I would put in more hot water. Sometimes when I got out of the bath, my heart would start pounding ... no doubt I'd overdone it with the water temperature.

I could go for a walk in 35°C weather wearing a heavy sweater, or in −30°C wearing short sleeves. It wasn't the outside temperature dictating what I wore, but my brain — my internal autistic structure.

This doesn't mean that you shouldn't advise someone to dress warmly! We must remember that the body necessarily reacts to its environment and that it really is cold. If the work of cognitive organization isn't done, an autistic individual needs to be guided.

18. Why Do Autistic People Like Wearing Hoodies?

You often see autistic people wearing hoodies. One of our hypotheses in this book is that autistic individuals find it hard to move around in space and time because of the particular wiring of their brain. They always need to be aware of the contours of the body in order to help their nervous system, which does not work smoothly. This phenomenon is often confused with proprioception issues, but the latter are quite different from the real problems caused by autism.

Autistic people will therefore often help themselves by wearing this kind of clothing because it gives them a uniform feel that follows the contours of their body and sends them a continuous, regular image of it. This frees the brain to do its work.

> When you see someone wearing clothing like this, remind yourself that it's not a whim but rather something the person needs for a stable reference point. Don't force them to take it off without giving them the help they need to get their bearings.

Autistic people often wear caps, headbands, or a pair of headphones with a band as a protective measure that helps them to maintain their stability. A particular area of the head seems to be the location of a mechanism that manages autistic brain structure. When this mechanism is destabilized, we see autistic people hitting their heads to try to stop the physical sensation inside.

> Be careful when you ask an autistic person to take off whatever they are wearing on their head.

19. Why Is He So Picky About Clothes?

Why does my child always want to wear the same clothes? He refuses to wear jeans, for example, and it's hard to get him to wear new clothes. The parent often has to wash the orange sweater while the child is sleeping, because that's the only thing he will want to wear

Brigitte: Autistic people come up with their own survival tactics. For example, we choose to wear long or baggy clothes so that people can't touch us without our seeing it. This means that we won't be disturbed by extra information to process that would simply add to the constant work of locating ourselves, and might interfere with it.

When someone touches me, my brain needs to perceive the touch and register it visually, otherwise it can't make the link between what I feel and what I see. I will stay blocked with the "imprint" of this touch for hours, while my whole brain has to try to analyze this touch. It's very unpleasant.

If an autistic person is reluctant to let his head be touched, that's why. The head is the central console where everything is controlled manually, on the inside. Wearing a hood provides a stable reference. Wearing a cap or a headband allows the individual to manage things better.

when he wakes up. It's impossible to persuade him to wear anything else!

Because the autistic brain only processes one piece of information at a time, it has difficulty processing several textures and/or colours at the same time. Autistic people don't care about fashion, so they don't choose clothes the same way neurotypical people do. Instead, they choose their clothes to help them manage their autism — clothes that will give them the smallest number of information fragments to process on a cognitive level. This is a survival mechanism.

In addition, for some autistic people, certain articles of clothing are directly associated with particular

Neurotypical thinking: interactive, having a global overview. The brain is dynamic and makes something "new."

Autistic thinking: associative, not drawing on previous experience. The brain is static; it associates or combines things.

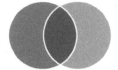
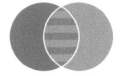

Figure 4: Neurotypical thinking compared with autistic thinking

activities or contexts. In order to process information, the autistic brain is excellent at making associations, but it is less good at organizing and synthesizing (Figure 4). An autistic person might wear certain pants for travelling to school and take them off when they get there, because it's impossible to get them to wear clothes perceived as having a different function or being for a different occasion. Once the link is made between school and a certain item of clothing, it's often difficult, or even impossible, for the person to change it. They need help to do things differently.

> Autistic people respond to their interior needs — the needs of their manual brain. This is not a whim. We need to be patient with them; when the cognitive organization is done, they will be able to make a variety of choices.

Brigitte: During the period when I was trying to decode my environment, I had to wear a particular bodysuit that covered my whole body. The garment was completely uniform: the fact of wearing one item of clothing with the same texture on my whole body meant I only had to notice a single thing; I could put any item of clothing over it if I was going out. My brain refused to process clothing made of two different fabrics or textures — that would have been one variable too many. By wearing this layer, I was able to dress appropriately for every situation, especially for work.

Since I had managed to recognize the texture of one item of clothing all over my body, with identical material everywhere, I was able to imagine this material in relation to my body as it moved. Later on, I was able to decode individual articles of clothing visually. However, I only wore one colour, because it was very taxing for my brain to notice two or more colours. So I've dressed in blue from head to toe for many years. I am just starting to be able to associate the image of my clothes with their texture — the texture is what I connect with my body and my movements through space.

Having clothes of the same colour allows me to move more easily without my eyes needing to constantly check my clothes. My head can focus on other things more easily if there is only one visual element to process.

When I started doing conference tours in the early 2000s, I had to sleep in many different hotel rooms. I had to pack huge pyjamas with a hood that I wore at night, so I wouldn't have to decode all those new beds with their sheets, pillows, colours, and so on. Sleeping in my big pyjamas protected me from the multiple exhausting mental identifications that would otherwise have been necessary, and I managed to sleep. I had solved the problem in a very simple way!

20. Why Do Autistic People Need So Much Time to Get Going in the Morning?

We often reproach autistic people for taking too long to get going in the morning, or accuse them of dragging out their preparations for school or work. An autistic individual is always short of time, even if she is convinced she's hurrying. From the outside, it might look as though she's waiting for a green light to get going with her activities.

For a lot of autistic people, the brain starts up slowly in the morning because of the burden of the manoeuvres that need to be done consciously. This phenomenon is most evident in people who are less in need of being told what to do, one action at a time. Because they can now do some things automatically, the process is quicker — but it still requires a lot of things to be learned by heart, and they have to work hard to get the cognitive mechanism going manually. This is slow and laborious.

Managing the autistic brain is complex. The autistic person must consciously follow several steps one after the other as she makes progress. For example, a young autistic woman has listed the different steps that she has to go through every morning when she wakes up: push off the covers, get out of bed, walk to the wardrobe, take her clothes out, switch off the night light, go to the window, grasp and pull the curtain, make the bed, go to the door, leave the room …

For a neurotypical person, the morning routine can be summarized much more quickly, because many of the steps have become automatic and don't require as much conscious effort as the autistic person needs to put in.

> *Brigitte:* A few years ago, I decided that from that point on I would get up at five in the morning to be ready to function around seven. That way I could manage to get ready for the day. Otherwise, my morning routine would be too fast for me: when I wake up, my brain needs about two hours of warming up before it is synchronized with my environment. Because it's hard to get going any more quickly, I made the decision to sleep less — but to be less stressed in the mornings by the pressure to go more quickly.

We need to be sure to give autistic people enough time in the mornings to get the day started. It's pointless rushing an autistic person and asking her to hurry up; this only creates more anxiety. Ultimately, when the necessary cognitive organization work is complete, she will reach a more fluid level of information processing that will allow her to speed up her routine at the start of the day.

21. Why Is Sleep So Hard for Autistic People?

Why can't he sleep, or only sleep a little? How is it that he can manage to fall asleep at night, but if he wakes up in the night he can't go back to sleep and even feels ready to start the day? Why does a parent have to sleep with their child if they want to get any sleep themselves?

Sleep problems are often associated with autism, and do seem to be caused by it. Several factors can cause a lack of sleep, including the inability to notice tiredness or a need for sleep, even if the person falls asleep quickly because their body is tired. The body is doing its work, but the brain doesn't receive the information. Autistic people cannot wait until they realize they are tired to go to bed. They need an evening routine. Another factor might be the many images from the day that the mind hasn't sorted out yet. At bedtime, you should avoid telling autistic children overly complex stories so as not to give them even more images to sort out. They are likely to spend the whole night doing it! If you tell them a story, it should be very short, with a visual accompaniment. You can also just draw their day with them.

The lack of a concept of time also plays an important role. The autistic child who wakes up in the middle of the night might not know that the night isn't over. As soon as

Lise: Without an understanding of time, we can't fully understand the concepts of "day" and "night." For autistic people, everything happens in real time. With no ability to notice tiredness, and without a real concept of time that gives meaning to day and night, how could they understand that it's time to sleep? A brain that doesn't process abstract information cannot understand the idea of sleeping alone or the absence of others ("Where do other people go while I'm sleeping?"). An autistic person finds himself in the dark and doesn't know when it will be light again! It's therefore vital to give him indications and explanations that he can understand, for example using a night light.

his eyes are open, he's ready to get up and play, whatever time it is. It is therefore essential to provide external visual clues that indicate the start and end of the night.

The bedroom of an autistic person should not be rearranged while they are sleeping; otherwise, they will have to start decoding again when they wake up. Sometimes parents put objects back in their children's rooms while they sleep, or put clean clothes on their dresser — this changes the room's configuration and can upset the child when he or she wakes up.

Putting the bed along the wall can significantly help an autistic child to sleep. Whenever possible, put the bed along the wall when the child is present, and allow her to take the new information in before going to sleep.

Brigitte: I used to live by the rhythm of external references. I went to bed because it was ten thirty. I spent sleepless nights because I wasn't tired. I couldn't feel my tiredness. Ever since I was young, I've preferred to read at night because I thought that lying down doing nothing was a complete waste of time. I could have been doing so many things! I knew I was going to bed just because it was nighttime.

As an adult, I didn't understand what I was doing in bed with my eyes open, trying to sleep. I knew I was tired after working for forty hours and one second, because my psychologist had told me that I was tired after forty hours of hard work! And when I did feel tired, it was so overwhelming that I almost passed out.

It's important to respect the internal functioning of an autistic person and give her regular breaks throughout the day. Since she is constantly bombarded with new information, she tires more quickly than neurotypical people. We can't wait to take a break until she's exhausted, nor wait for her to tell us she needs to rest, since she can detect only extreme fatigue. A break consists of a structured sequence with a beginning and an end and doesn't include any stimulation, including electronic screens.

5

Learning

22. Is It True That Autistic People Need Routines?

➤ **Myth: Autistic people need routines.**

We read everywhere that autistic people need actions to be repeated, the same thing in the same order, otherwise there's a crisis. For example, if you're going to Grandma's house, you always have to drive the same way, otherwise the autistic person will lose their bearings.

We need to look at the "need" for fixed routines from a different angle. Autistic people's brains create links by what can be seen, that is, from the outside or in the surrounding environment, rather than on the inside, in the mind. A fixed route allows the introduction of a static, stabilizing element amid the flow of information coming in. Remember that the autistic brain only processes what it knows.

Brigitte: When your reference points are all external, life is not simple: the idea of time is very different. My routine consisted of eating at set hours, having lunch at noon on the dot. If the phone rang at 11:57, it was a catastrophe and I had a surge of anxiety: what if I answered and the call lasted more than three minutes — I wouldn't be able to eat!

An autistic person therefore needs some routines. But their obsessive routine-seeking is associated with information processing — it's not deliberate and it is not related to inflexibility.

With the help of a tool like SACCADE Conceptual Language, an autistic person can start to process incoming information more fluidly and to avoid artificial routines created for the sake of information processing. Like everyone else, autistic people need to have routines — without going overboard.

23. Why Do Autistic People Always Watch the Same Films? Why Do They Want to Watch the Same Film or the Same Scene Dozens of Times, No Matter How Old They Are?

Autistic people are social creatures, just like all humans: they are constantly seeking meaning, including the meaning of social interactions. A high-functioning autistic individual will watch the same film several times to go over particular social scenes, to analyze and understand them. Since we can't stop people in the street and

> *Brigitte:* I've watched a huge number of films in my life. Since I've never been able to ask people to repeat what they've just said or ask them for help figuring out what they mean, films helped me. I would get home in the evening and choose a film that had a scene I knew could help me. Then I could take the time to analyze it and try to understand what had happened. Since I knew my films off by heart, I could quickly choose the scene I needed!
>
> Being "socially blind" means not being able to follow social exchanges as they happen — the task is too complex. When more than four people were talking around me, it was like trying to follow a hockey game with an invisible puck: I could never see where the shot came from, but I could see who received the pass!

interrogate them about their behaviour (there's no remote control for people!), it's easier for an autistic person to research social meaning in films, where they can control the viewing experience.

For a more severely affected individual, watching the same film scenes over and over is associated with the brain's need to process a known, continuous movement. Some people even start with the opening credits, because they resemble a page to be read from top to bottom, which is easier for the perceptive brain. This is a developmental stage of autism.

An autistic person needs to watch a film several times before they can fully grasp it. Before they get to the emotion the film might provoke, they have to analyze all the twists and turns of the plot in detail. That way they register each of the film's images one by one, which can take a long time.

> We must be patient and allow an autistic person to watch a film as many times as she wants. The individual will use every means available to try to make progress. She is intelligent, therefore she seeks meaning.

24. He Speaks; He's Intelligent: Does He Need Visual Clues?

People often tell us that an autistic friend or family member doesn't need any visual aids (for example pictograms, words, or short passages of text) because he can speak, is intelligent, and understands them when they speak to him.

Using visual aids effectively helps the individual organize cognition in an integrated way. In fact, an autistic person's brain behaves to some extent as if the person were deaf or blind, with one sense compensating for another. In this case, the visual compensates.

This visual compensation has nothing to do with speech or intelligence. Most autistic people speak. Saying that an autistic individual doesn't speak is like saying that a deaf person is mute. The deaf person's speech delay is caused by their deafness; the speech delay of an autistic person is caused by the brain's wiring. If there are no other problems, the autistic person will speak when they reach the appropriate stage of development.

We shouldn't hesitate to present visual aids to an autistic person, whatever their age. Not using visual aids would be like avoiding sign language around a person who is hard of hearing.

The visual aspect is part of communication. If a person visits a country where she does not speak the language, her first instinct will be to use pictures and gestures, or to get out pen and paper to communicate by drawing. We would say that such a person is resourceful and independent, even though we know perfectly well that she can express herself verbally.

> It's vital to support communication with visual aids because they allow autistic people to organize their thoughts and to incorporate information in the long term. Whatever the degree to which they are affected, autistic people understand and think in pictures. Visual aids give meaning, especially to things that are invisible or abstract. Remember that when an autistic individual is anxious, the visual channel is the only one that operates. A support person should always have a pen and paper within reach.

25. Do All Autistic People Need Pictograms?

➤ Myth: All autistic people need pictograms.

Some people believed that it was necessary to show a lot of pictograms to autistic people. This is untrue. Other people thought the opposite: that it was pointless to show pictograms to autistic children — that it might do them harm, or infantilize them, or stop them from speaking. In any case, if the children did what was asked of them, what would be the benefit of introducing pictograms?

If pictograms are used well, they can be abandoned after a while. This stage of visual conceptualization is

Even though pictograms can support conceptualization by allowing the individual to interact with the environment, they aren't the only aids required, because they are static and must be accompanied by conceptual tools. To solve this problem, we created SACCADE Conceptual Language (SCL), a graphic code that is more effective than pictograms and can increase the quality of life of autistic people.

SCL is a transition tool that helps autistic people reach "independent linguistic mode": in other words, becoming verbal. It helps build an individual's cognitive organization by getting around the brain's inability to self-start, improves the capacity for abstract thinking, and reduces the delay in information processing, which gives access to the self in real time. It helps make the brain flexible and reduces rituals, echolalia, and significant stereotyped behaviour; in doing this, it helps autistic people move on to a different stage of development.

Created by an autistic person, SCL follows the stages of autistic development. It's a more natural language for autistic people and has an effect on the cognitive structure itself. We believe that a language for autistic people should be adaptable for use with everyone on the spectrum and not target people of just one degree of severity, so that all have access to real communication. SCL is suited to autistic people of all degrees of severity: a severely affected adult or two-year-old, a higher-functioning four-year-old or thirty-year-old engineer.

essential, but seems not to get started by itself in autistic people. This developmental stage has nothing to do with the ability to speak.

Our understanding of how to use pictograms is flawed. Pictograms are supposed to help an autistic person to understand concepts visually, with the aim of helping them become more verbal. Many people base their analysis on neurotypical functioning rather than autistic functioning, so they have trouble understanding the real usefulness of these tools.

Every autistic individual needs visual conceptualization, but they don't necessarily need pictograms. Visual tools, if they are used well, should help autistic people increase their abilities in conceptualization, abstraction, and comprehension.

When autistic people reject pictograms, it's because they have progressed in their development. They have passed that stage. However, that certainly does not mean that they no longer need to conceptualize visually.

26. What Is the Difference Between Autism Spectrum Disorder (ASD) and Intellectual Disability?

➤ Myth: Autism is a kind of intellectual disability.

For a long time, autism was confused with intellectual disability. Even a few years ago, people were offering up statistics to suggest that 75 percent of autistic people also had an intellectual disability. Today, that figure has dropped to 25 percent, and some studies report an even lower number.

Because of these incorrect data, many inappropriate therapeutic choices are still being made as if autistic people automatically had an intellectual disability. Many autism services are established based on existing services for people with intellectual difficulties. This is a serious mistake.

We must remember that autistic people have a different cognitive organization; if we see signs of intellectual disability, that is a separate issue. Services must therefore be adapted to match the reality of autistic cognitive organization. It's easy to fall into the trap of offering maintenance services rather than services that respect the individual developing brain. We must also be cautious when it comes to criteria for measuring intellectual disability. Being "socially blind" does not mean that a person has an intellectual disability.

We once worked with an autism professional who showed us a client profile: a young man of fourteen, an autistic boy with a moderate intellectual disability who loved math and whose favourite TV program was Radio-Canada's scientific discovery program. How could a person show an interest in science and have a moderate intellectual disability? If you don't understand autism, you won't understand the autistic individual.

Autism involves different brain wiring from that of a neurotypical person. We must take the time to learn about it before concluding that an autistic individual has reached their developmental ceiling. We must also be careful when talking about developmental ceilings. An autistic person might simply be on the verge of total exhaustion, especially because their over-connected brain demands a lot of energy to process additional incoming information. The danger, in therapy, is not allowing the autistic person enough time to reach their full potential.

> Be observant: a human being cannot have a part-time intellectual disability!

27. Why Do Autistic People Always Ask the Same Questions?

At a particular developmental stage, an autistic person might repeat the same questions over and over again. For example, they might ask "When are we going to the movie?" several times a day for several days.

It doesn't matter how many times you, the adult, reply in every way you can think of ("We're going on Saturday," "We're going in four days," "You know when, it's the usual time," etc.); the questioning never ends. More intriguing still, the child can give the exact same answer to the question if you ask her. So why does she constantly repeat the same question?

For a visual brain, a verbal answer is not an answer, it's something without meaning, sounds that have not yet become related to a meaning. And things without meaning cause anxiety.

When an autistic person keeps asking the same question, it might be that he is stuck and can't grasp the answer, even if he is intelligent, and is trying to figure out what it means. It can also indicate that there is work to be done on the cognitive organization front so that sounds become meaningful words.

We must respond visually, situating the information in time if need be. "When?" "In three sleeps." Get out your pen and paper, quick! Use the same vocabulary if you can. Don't forget that the information given in reply must be clear, precise, and matched to the person's level of understanding. Speak more slowly if necessary.

28. Why Do Autistic People Always Say "I Don't Know" to Questions?

"When I ask questions like 'How are you?' or 'What did you have for breakfast?' the answer is always the same: 'I don't know.' But he can speak, and has a lot of impressive knowledge. I know full well that he is intelligent, so why does he always say 'I don't know'?"

This is a very common answer from autistic people.

One of the three characteristics common to autistic people is the difficulty in recalling information. Autistic people can't quickly call to mind the images associated with an experience, even if it was recent.

At the moment she says "I don't know," she is being totally honest. It's not a joke. She needs visual help to reduce the delay in processing information. Without it, the only way she can answer a question about what she did earlier is "I don't know" — and she's right!

Autistic people are not cut off from reality, but they are cut off from the meaning of things and the coherence of the world. They need to be helped to make links. An answer like "I don't know" indicates that there is still cognitive organization work to be done.

Brigitte: If an autistic person says "I don't know" to me, this is valuable information. I used to say the same thing for years when people asked me about my life. The reason for this was very simple: every time I tried to answer that kind of question, my brain didn't know where to go! The immediate environment was very clear for me, but when I tried to access my personal experience, it was as if I needed a GPS to get to where my lived experiences were stored. My "internal telescope" seemed to be in a huge black room and I didn't know where to aim it. Later on, I learned that I had to explore this black space to find answers. Using SACCADE Conceptual Language, I constructed a building, room by room, that allows me to access this information a little more easily today.

6

Self-Esteem

29. Should Autistic People Try to Broaden Their Interests?

It's often said that autistic people have very specific and narrow interests, for example numbers, letters, dinosaurs, bus or train timetables, geography, ancient history.

In treatment plans, workers will often suggest that the client try to broaden their interests. The fact that the autistic person is deeply committed to a particular subject seems to bother the people around her. But why is it that a neurotypical person who's really interested in flowers has a wonderful passion and is valued? Nobody around her would ever think that she should find other interests. So why do we try to modify the interests of autistic people?

> People's interests are part of them. They correspond to their perceptions, their desires, and their talents. We should not try to discourage them.

The autistic person will find other interests as they progress to higher developmental stages, which will give them more breadth. Working on conceptualization will allow this to happen. Narrow interests are a result of the way the perceptive brain processes information. By making the information processing more fluid, we can help individuals to diversify their interests — if they want to.

For autistic people, specific interests develop "inside" the wider field. Because the brain can only make concrete links, the person will develop a deep interest through exploring all the details.

For example, if someone is interested in trains, she will be interested in different types of trains, different periods of train history, the countries in which they are built, railways, the screws and bolts used, timetables, and so on.

30. Do They Have Emotions?

➤ **Myth: Autistic people don't feel emotions.**

Observers have long believed that autistic people don't feel emotion. What a mistake!

Reading the emotions of autistic people is more complicated than it might seem. One thing is certain: all humans have emotions, including autistic people. But some myths last a long time.

We must remember that the map of primary emotions is the same as for neurotypical people. There's fear, anger, sadness, and joy. But since the brain understands information differently, the triggers for these emotions are different from those of neurotypical people. These triggers are directly related to the experiences of autistic people.

What makes an autistic person laugh won't necessarily make a neurotypical person laugh. Because of their perceptive brains, autistic people might laugh at a toy's physical imperfections; a neurotypical person might laugh at seeing the toy hit another toy, for example. And autistic individuals don't show emotion in the same ways as neurotypical people.

Because the autistic brain has to pass through various developmental stages, some autistic people won't cry at certain stages; others won't yet be able to express the emotions they feel. You need to know autism to understand how emotions develop, since the way they are expressed depends on the developmental stage of the individual.

Unfortunately, these emotional expressions can be misinterpreted as problematic, especially for those around the autistic person. An angry autistic person is not a person with behaviour problems, but simply an angry human being. He merely uses different signals to express that same anger. The emotions of autistic individuals are identical to those of others; only their expression is different.

You can be sure that an autistic person who cries is in pain, one who laughs is experiencing happiness, one who shows signs of anger is genuinely feeling anger, and one who seems afraid really is afraid.

When it comes to the emotions of autistic people, you can't pretend to be a specialist. It's important to not treat the autistic person as neurotypical, which can do more harm than good.

31. What Should We Tell Friends and Family About Autism?

Friends and family might ask, "Are you sure he's autistic? He doesn't seem like it. He doesn't look autistic!" In our field, we know that the less visible the autism is, the more difficult it is to explain, because the real explanation lies in the brain's wiring, which can't be seen. Some people may think they have cured an individual because they no longer observe autistic symptoms.

Would we think of saying that a deaf person has a behavioural problem because she doesn't answer to her name? Would we say that a blind person has a behavioural problem if she refuses to cross the road because she doesn't have all the information she needs to be safe?

Autism is neither an illness nor a behavioural problem but a neurodevelopmental disorder. The autistic brain is visual and concrete. When we use only words to communicate with an autistic person, he might not understand everything fully — words, at that moment, might not be enough. Autistic mental representations involve images and associations. We might think he is choosing not to hear, but that is not the case.

He is intelligent and he can speak. But he is cut off from the meaning of social interactions, from abstraction. We need to help by showing him the meaning that he can't perceive because he can't see it with his eyes. No, this is not voluntary, and his parents are not to blame. Yes, this can cause him a great deal of anxiety. And yes, he will develop if we help him by using a neurodevelopmental approach that responds to his autistic brain's needs.

> To sum up, this is what you should say to people close to an autistic individual: Autism is a neurodevelopmental problem that affects development for a person's whole life. The wiring of the autistic brain is different from that of a neurotypical brain. It's normal not to notice immediately that a person has autism. More than 1 percent of the world's population is on the autism spectrum.

Brigitte: The neurotypical brain comes with automatic gears. It receives and processes information smoothly because it has reliable automatic settings (the strategies it has learned and has easy access to) and can therefore work on several tasks at the same time. It's not really aware of the information processing, which happens quickly and without deliberate thought. But an autistic person has a brain with manual transmission. Every piece of information that comes in has to be treated on its own, and with great effort. An autistic person must be allowed enough time to carry out these manoeuvres.

32. Is It True That All Autistic People Are Aggressive?

➤ **Myth: Autistic people are aggressive.**

False! Aggressiveness is not a characteristic of autism. However, many autistic people are unintentionally besieged by those around them and by their environment. Autistic people are aggressed by people who talk too much, or who talk and touch at the same time, by continual gaps in meaning, by people interfering because they don't understand autism, by treatments that have been imposed on autistic people that they didn't ask for, etc.

In short, if they are aggressed and **unable** to react, and if they are blocked and aren't getting help to manage their autism, people might become aggressive. However, we often say that an aggressive autistic person is an aggressed person who doesn't really mean to be aggressive.

We need to understand that autistic people are in survival mode. While others are trying to make her appear neurotypical or "socially acceptable," to make her particularities or her movements disappear, the autistic individual is simply trying to survive.

33. Why Is She So Anxious?

We are often asked why autistic people are so anxious. She can speak, she's intelligent, but she's so anxious! Medication doesn't seem to control her anxiety. What is going on?

Autistic people are constantly wrestling with their

condition. Despite their intelligence, autistic people have to deal with a "manual brain" that often gets stuck while trying to "manually" adapt to new information. The autistic brain is under-connected in terms of communication, which prevents the individual from expressing himself the way he wants. Caught between internal and external demands, trying to process a dynamic environment with his static brain, he experiences a great deal of anxiety and wears himself out trying to stay balanced.

The level of anxiety that an autistic person feels is a good indicator of the work that still needs to be done on cognitive organization. But he can't do this work alone; he needs help. Medication won't work in this situation because this anxiety is specific to autism and different from social anxiety. Usually, working with SACCADE Conceptual Language allows him to reduce the anxiety and give meaning and coherence to the information he takes in.

Brigitte: I was always anxious without knowing why. Nor did I know that I was different from other people: I had to be taught that. Some autistic people are able to see their differences very quickly, while others learn about them from others.

Today, I see that I have always had to work very hard in a world that moves far too quickly for me. The anxiety from managing the autism was more severe than the anxiety I had in social situations. From the moment I woke up in the morning, the effort I had to make to get through the day, combined with the difficulties of being autistic, was enormous. I became burned out and suicidal before I was thirty because I didn't know that I had to manage my autism every day.

7

Social Skills

➤ **Myth: If she has a sense of humour, she can't be autistic.**

How many times have we heard people say things like "This person can't be on the autism spectrum: she makes jokes!"

Autistic people have a sense of humour too. But since their frame of reference is different (it's non-social), their humour will be different too: more perceptive than social.

When a neurotypical person notices that an autistic person is laughing for no apparent reason, he's right: what an autistic person finds funny flies right over the head of a neurotypical person, and vice versa. Neurotypical people will laugh about a social irregularity (for example, if it is pointed out by a comedian), while autistic people laugh about perceptive irregularities.

> *Brigitte:* When parents tell me their autistic children's jokes, in groups where everyone is neurotypical, I am often the only person to laugh, because our humour is very different from that of other people. It's based on our concrete and perceptive frame of reference. The neurotypical individuals who spread the myth that autistic people have no sense of humour must have been pretty miserable! Today, I tell people who say that "autistic people laugh for no apparent reason" that they're right: they can't see the reason because they have a neurotypical brain!

What is a perceptive irregularity? It could be a row of light bulbs where one of them is broken. Or just the sound of a word. While these things might make someone on the autism spectrum laugh, a neurotypical person will wonder what's so funny.

A sense of humour, like every other emotional trigger, is filtered through the autistic brain.

35. Does He Love Me?

➤ **Myth: Autistic people are unable to love neurotypical people.**

The studies are unequivocal: autistic people form attachments. Any expert will tell you that she has observed an autistic individual getting on well with his family members. But he won't express his attachment in the same way. Someone with a more severe degree of autism might touch his mother's hair and flap his hands with joy to show that he recognizes her.

It takes unprejudiced observation to understand the attachments and emotions of autistic people. The period when we thought that autistic people had no emotions and couldn't form attachments to people — and that this was the parents' fault — has left many scars.

Today, because of magnetic resonance imaging, our picture of the autistic brain is getting better and better. We know enough to understand that autistic characteristics are biological, not emotional, in nature. But many people still confuse autism and attachment issues.

When an autistic person has reached a certain level of maturity, she can concretely demonstrate her attachment. Would we expect a baby a few weeks old to concretely demonstrate attachment? No, because we are well aware that he is in the process of creating that bond. Since autism is a neurodevelopmental issue, the brain must be given time to reach a sufficient level of awareness.

Those who try to teach autistic people to say "I love you" are merely satisfying the needs of neurotypical people. An autistic child is simply learning to repeat the sound, which is still empty of meaning for him at this stage. You could teach him to say "rhinoceros" and it would mean the same thing. When the child is ready, saying "I love you" will come by itself, without an external command. The work done to develop the autistic brain will bring this result about naturally. When it does, you will know that the expression of love is genuine, because it is fully understood, intentional, and felt. Today, mothers rush to tell us that they've had their first "I love you" without ever having done any work to achieve it.

36. What Is a Tantrum? What Is an
    Autistic Crisis?

➤ **Myth: All autistic people have tantrums or meltdowns; behaviour modification and punishments
are appropriate techniques for controlling these
outbursts.**

We hear every day about autistic people having tantrums
or meltdowns. We hear that they bang their heads, throw
themselves on the ground, bite their own hands or arms,
yell, cry, explode ... Before labelling this behaviour as a
tantrum or meltdown, we need to consider what is different about an autistic crisis.

In the current literature, there is nothing to say that
tantrums are related to the way the autistic brain works. It's
only from a non-autistic frame of reference that people have
decided that these are always anger tantrums. There are different levels of crisis for autistic people. The basic autistic
crisis is when the person is banging their head. There are
two clues for identifying a true autistic crisis: during it,
there are no tears, and afterwards, the person is exhausted.
This is a crisis related to autism and its concomitant brain
wiring issues rather than a tantrum resulting from anger.
What people perceive as a tantrum is actually a major
crisis, which is also caused by brain wiring issues, but is
even stronger.

These crises often express an attempt to understand a
complex piece of information. They aren't actually anger —
more like an internal storm or an earthquake, as if the different parts of the brain were not communicating with one

Brigitte: People who don't know much about autism mix up tantrums and crises. For years I've tried to pin down the precise emotion that brings about a crisis, the one that sets off a storm in the brain when it can't process some complex piece of information. I finally realized it was fear. When people don't distinguish between the two types of crisis, they end up punishing autistic people for being afraid.

another. These crises are involuntary and very upsetting for the person experiencing them.

It's important to differentiate between autistic crises and anger tantrums to avoid affecting self-esteem, particularly in so-called high-functioning autistic people.

Autistic crises are extremely exhausting for autistic people. It is pointless to try to stop the crisis by intervening physically — this will only make things worse. It's equally pointless to try to stop the person's movement, or to try to control the crisis by imitating it, which is a method used with people with behavioural difficulties. It would be unthinkable to say to a person with epilepsy, "If you don't have a seizure today, you can have a treat!" The same goes for autistic people. First and foremost, we need to consider the autistic brain, putting aside our neurotypical expectations and interpretations.

Crises are an involuntary cry for help, since the autistic person can't seek help by themselves, no matter their age, because their communication channel is affected. It is our duty to help autistic people find the equilibrium they need and to support their brain development.

There's just one thing to remember: during the crisis, stay silent while making sure the person doesn't injure themselves.

37. Is He Manipulating Me?

"He's just having a tantrum ... I tell you, if that was my child ...!"

People have been led to believe that autistic children manipulate adults, that they use tantrums, that they know very well what they should be doing but refuse, and so on. Parents and caregivers often hear such hurtful comments, which don't match their lived reality. Parents are well placed to know whether a child is manipulating them or not, and often find themselves caught between autistic behaviour that they don't understand and other people's judgment.

We now know that the autistic brain isn't capable of making inferences. It imitates behaviours but not intentions. It doesn't produce or comprehend subtext. It can't position its own emotions in space and time, let alone other people's.

To be able to manipulate someone, you need to figure out what they are thinking and lead them to change their mind without their agreement and by means of precise actions. An autistic person can't do this without developing a capacity for abstract thought and reading social situations. On the other hand, a person on the autism spectrum can try to provoke a reaction in you just to see the reaction, the same way a young child would.

When you hear someone say "Are you sure? She doesn't look autistic!" you are colliding with other people's ignorance. What does "looking autistic" even mean? Most people don't understand what autism is, but they think they know something about it because they've seen *Rain Man*.

Trust your instinct when it comes to reading your child: if he seems distressed, it's because he is distressed. If he cries, it means he's sad. His distress is often caused by other people's lack of understanding. If he's stuck, and someone carries on harassing him, he will become aggressive too. If we punished a deaf person because he couldn't hear, we wouldn't be surprised if he became aggressive, depressed, or suicidal.

When your child does develop the ability to manipulate you, remind yourself that this is an excellent sign! That means that she has made progress.

38. Why Aren't Autistic People Interested in Socializing?

How many times have you wished an autistic person you know would come to a party, an event, or a social gathering? How many times has that person declined such an invitation? In general, autistic people don't like being around lots of other people.

The specific wiring of the autistic brain prioritizes patterns and images. These are concentrated on the brain's perceptive side, which means that the brain is primarily interested in precise information, details, and concrete things, and is less interested in abstract — and therefore social — things.

Brigitte: At work I heard someone say you ought to call your friends every two weeks if you wanted to keep them. I had to make myself lots of reminders that I stuck around my office, near my phone, to remind me to phone the friends I didn't want to lose. Then I realized one day that I had been a friend to a lot of people, in the sense that I had made a lot of gestures of friendship, but that I had never actually had a lot of friends myself. The social obligations I was trying to maintain demanded a lot of energy and I didn't always understand why they were necessary. It wasn't natural — they were simply tasks I had learned off by heart. So I decided to radically prune my social life so that I wouldn't end up giving up on it altogether. I took a break for a while because I couldn't carry on. Even today, I find this kind of management too complex and demanding for me.

As far as social interactions are concerned, an autistic person "doesn't know what she doesn't know" because her brain is "socially blind." We must not confuse autism with being emotionally cut off from social life. They are two very different things. Many autistic people like other people once they can understand them. Our observations are now validated by research using cerebral imaging, autistic voices, and our own experiences in working with autistic people, which show us that many are very interested in being social once they can manage to process information about social situations.

Do not trust programs that seek to teach social skills too soon to autistic people. Autism is a neurodevelopmental disorder, and we must respect the individual's development above all else. If the person hasn't yet reached the stage of development where socializing is possible, it's pointless to insist that she learn these skills, which will merely cause further anxiety. Would we try to teach a nine-month-old baby how to make friends because we thought he ought to know that already? Of course not! We would wait for the right developmental stage. The same goes for autistic people.

39. Why Don't Autistic People Want to Shake Hands?

You will often notice that an autistic person won't spontaneously offer to shake hands in greeting. Why is this?

When an autistic person is touched, his eyes look at the place where he was touched. If he shakes hands, his eyes go straight to the hands, which is not considered polite in Western society. In order to pull off this manoeuvre while seeming to be "socially acceptable," many autistic people invent little work-arounds.

Some people will have a fixed gaze because they are concentrating on locating the touch. Others always say the same phrase while looking at the other person's forehead.

Shaking an acquaintance's hand is completely unremarkable for a neurotypical person, but it's a small example of the social obligations that we impose on those who need to prioritize their own internal management to rebalance their perturbed system. Before you ask an autistic person to shake hands, think: Is it really necessary? For whom?

What does a handshake mean for an autistic person? First of all, she can't move — she has to stay still. Then she has to visually calculate the contact between the two hands. Once contact is made, she has to consciously lift her gaze to meet the other person's, or at least to look at their nose or forehead. Next, she has to look for an appropriate length of time. If the other person says something during the handshake, the autistic person will have to ask them to repeat it, since her brain can only process one piece of information at a time.

40. Should Autistic People Learn Social Behaviour, Such as Greetings, Off by Heart?

In Quebec we used to think that because autistic people had trouble with social skills, it was really important to teach those skills, to allow them to "fit in" socially. The vast majority ended up learning social skills by heart, which led to a belief that for autistic people, learning things off by heart was normal!

Teaching social skills betrays a major flaw in understanding autism, because learning things off by heart is not normal. Autism is a neurodevelopmental disorder. We have to wait for the autistic brain to reach a certain developmental stage before socialization becomes possible.

People who misunderstood autism thought we needed to teach social skills to people with social blindness. But they didn't consider the particular brain wiring involved. The methods that were used could only lead to social skills being learned off by heart.

Here's a classic example: Each morning as she walks into the classroom, the teacher says good morning to her pupil, who doesn't reply. She explains to him — verbally — that he ought to say good morning to her when she comes in. That day, the teacher goes out of the classroom four times, and every time she comes back in, the pupil says good morning to her. That lasts for the entire school year. Is that really what we want to achieve?

Today, we know that most autistic people will develop social skills without having to learn them off by heart. And there are specific ways of supporting their development.

41. He Doesn't Look at Me. Should I Force Him to Make Eye Contact?

➤ **Myth: He won't look at me while I'm speaking, so he's not listening to me.**

In the literature, much is said about the fact that autistic people won't make eye contact when they're talking to someone. People have tried to intervene by forcing eye contact, believing that once it was established, it would lead to something further — as with social skills.

They were on the wrong track. When we interview autistic people, we observe that it is cruel to force them to make eye contact. While it might comfort the neurotypical person, it does nothing for the autistic person. Children will learn to establish eye contact in order to please neurotypical people, but this is not a long-lasting lesson, merely an extra chore people demand of them.

Brigitte: Other people's eyes move too quickly for me. On good days, they look like coloured marbles surrounded by white. Neurotypical people see the eyes as a way of knowing a person's mind. But I can't hold someone's gaze. And if my brain won't give me access to my own emotions, how could I read other people's through their eyes?

Once again: an autistic person is socially blind. Other people's eyes are not a way for me to figure out how they're feeling. If I want to know how someone is doing, I will ask him. And too bad for him if he doesn't tell me the truth! In any case, if he lies, with all his neurotypical communication abilities, he isn't respecting me as an autistic person. So I don't see why I should have to demonstrate more empathy than him!

Imposing eye contact on autistic people results from misunderstanding the way autism works and shows a total lack of respect. The autistic person is guided not by the gaze of the other but by her need to make sense of her surroundings.

We need to respect human development. First of all, an autistic person needs to look at the speaker's mouth to "see" the sound come out; visual contact will follow.

Remember that some studies have found a link between autistic brain wiring and social development.

8

Self-Regulation

12. Why Does an Intelligent Person on the Autism Spectrum, Someone with a Great Deal of Skill and Knowledge, Have Trouble Holding Down a Job?

Now that autistic people have degrees and can land jobs, it's unbelievable that they can't manage to keep them! What's going on?

If the necessary cognitive organization work hasn't been done, even an adult with a degree won't have the necessary initiative to handle the constant little adjustments needed to adapt to a changing environment. Since it has difficulty being flexible, the autistic brain can't plan ahead, which, without the support that's needed, may cause lifelong problems.

It's not uncommon for autistic people to successfully complete college or university programs but be unable to keep a job. They then find themselves either unemployed or seriously underemployed.

The autistic brain structure affects the individual's initiative, but also her ability to access information in real time, which means that the ability to seek out solutions might be lacking even in individuals who have improved their problem-solving skills.

Another factor to take into account with adults who could become independent is their difficulty reading social cues. Those whose autism is less visible might never have received the support that would help them manage their autistic brain.

Autism is a disorder involving neural connections. Good luck trying to see those! Even the most skilled autistic people get exhausted living alone in an apartment or working, because experts decided to "teach" them social skills instead of teaching them to conceptualize. Real learning develops abstract thinking and can be taught using a conceptual language. Autistic people who learn to make deductions, instead of just applying learned social behaviour, can

Lise: Think of the adult who can't reach a conclusion from the facts presented to him or plan an action within a timeframe: this is because he didn't receive the help his autistic brain needed. He might have several university degrees, but he can't keep a job and ends up stacking shelves at the grocery store. One day he's hanging around in front of the dairy shelves, where there's just one litre of milk left, waiting for that last litre to be gone so he can refill the shelves. So he loses his job. He remains stuck with the autistic brain wiring that won't allow him to make deductions.

achieve a sense of balance and adjust better to daily life. As a result, their lives will have more meaning.

43. How Can We Help Her Become Independent?

> **Myth: She's autistic; she'll never be independent; I'll be responsible for her for life.**

Because autism has long been confused with intellectual disability, therapies have been designed in the same way as those used for people with intellectual disabilities. We talk a lot about developing the person's independence, with the aim of getting them to do tasks by themselves: making the bed, cooking a meal, getting groceries. But when it comes to autism, this independence is not what we should be focusing on to begin with.

Will he be able to live his own life? How will he get training? We must understand that for an autistic person, independence doesn't mean learning social skills but properly balancing the processing of information, which promotes the ability for abstraction, and initiative. First we need to focus on self-regulation and then on independence.

Remember that self-regulation starts with the necessary work of finding equilibrium and synchronizing the autistic brain, followed by cognitive organization. As long as this work remains undone, the person will not become independent. We can teach her many things from the outside, by rote, but if she can't access internal plans that allow her to transfer knowledge to different contexts in

Brigitte: When I became an independent adult, I went to live in an apartment and started working. I had to move several times for work. Every time I arrived in a new apartment, I couldn't get my bearings in the new location. The physical space had a configuration I couldn't figure out. It wasn't until years later that I realized that I'd often slept in the living room because I'd never managed to fully decode my bedroom.

After one such move, I often wore the same clothes. A month later, I noticed someone at work turn up wearing a sweater identical to one of mine. I started wondering where my sweater was, and then, suddenly, several other items of clothing whose existence I'd forgotten popped into my head. Where could they be? When I got home that evening, I succeeded in decoding my bedroom's physical space and discovered that it had a closet. When I opened it, I found all my missing clothes! Someone had helped me with the move and put them away in there. And I hadn't even known there was a closet by my bed because I hadn't yet figured out my new environment …

her life, these will just be useless facts that need to be hoarded desperately so that they can't escape — which means more anxiety. Such a person might well have impressive knowledge, but she will always need someone else to set her in motion.

To help an autistic person become independent, start by not doing everything for him. Guide him to discover things. He must experience life on his own. This does not mean you should let him do whatever he wants; he needs to be guided and to have the meanings of things explained.

44. Will My Child Be Able to Go to School?

School is the best place for a child on the autism spectrum, as long as she understands how she learns and why she is at school. Her future depends on education. Currently, no institution is perfectly adapted to the autistic brain's ways of learning. Therefore the best place for an autistic child is wherever she will learn the most and be comfortable. Since she will have her whole life to develop socially, we should concentrate first on learning.

Schools should look after an autistic child the same way they would look after a student in the class who is blind or hard of hearing. The child might well be intelligent and get good grades at school, but she still has an autistic brain: we can't afford to wait until she is suffering from anxiety before helping her.

If the autistic child is not developing or getting "results," instead of blaming him we should come back to the question of how to do things and what tools to use. There is no reason for him not to go to school unless he also has a health problem. But because the autistic brain's ways of learning are so little understood, autism frightens people. We therefore need to work on sensitivity and social education.

9

Good to Know

45. When Should My Autistic Child Start Getting Help? Should I Wait for Problems to Start?

➤ **Myth: Autistic children just need to be loved —
that's enough to get them through it.**

So often, we hear "The autism isn't very visible, should we wait to get help?" Why wait? Wait for what? For the autism to go away?

Answer: Get help immediately.

As soon as an ASD diagnosis has been made, you can begin working. Autism is a neurodevelopmental disorder — a particular way the brain is wired. There is no need to wait for external signs before taking action. ASD becomes apparent when the brain struggles to process incoming information.

Learning to find internal equilibrium in real time and then working on cognitive organization is a long, slow

Brigitte: Despite all my resources, I had to seek help at the age of twenty-eight. This work lasted for years.

process that needs to start early, even if everything seems to be going well. Time has shown us that this work won't happen by itself. Sooner or later, the autism will become visible, often accompanied by anxiety. If we want to help the individual develop rather than stay at the same stage, we should make sure that learning is ongoing.

Autism is a constant, ongoing reality that will affect the person regardless of the availability of experts and services. Autistic people must be supported at all times.

46. Should We Use Electronic Devices to "Cure" Autism?

In this era of omnipresent technology, everyone wants a concrete tool to help autistic people.

The advent of new devices such as tablets has shown that autistic people have aptitudes and abilities in terms of perception that have long been ignored; this confirms recent research.

These devices are very appealing because they are good babysitters, in the sense that they allow adults to take their children out a little more and worry less. This applies to parents of neurotypical children, too!

However, the biggest challenge with autism is to lead the individual toward social awareness, which devices can never do. These devices should be used for educational purposes for a defined period of time — a few minutes a day at most, as for any other child. Just because a child is learning something on a tablet doesn't mean that they will be able to transfer that learning elsewhere. Furthermore, to our knowledge, no study has demonstrated that technology can improve social interaction among autistic people.

Autism is a language issue. Learning needs to involve another person, because the autistic person is learning *for* the other person, in order to be able to communicate with him. We will never "cure" all the problems of the autistic brain if we only use computers and tablets.

Moreover, since the autistic brain is already skilled in perception, the use of devices must be approached with a great deal of caution, so as not to reinforce what the autistic brain already does very well. The autistic person will not want to give up her device, with which she feels completely at ease, but other problems will appear. For example, some studies have shown that overuse of computer technology can affect sleep cycles, especially in neurotypical children.

> We need to be careful when it comes to screens! Because autistic people already work so hard processing the information that comes in, they need the chance to play sports or be physically active to spread out their energy expenditure over the day. The use of devices for leisure should be supervised.

Brigitte: I love electronic devices. I find them far less complicated than people and they are so useful for learning. But I came to realize that I couldn't learn social skills by practising with a device. Human exchanges and emotions are very different in real life. It's important for me to make an effort to be with people, so I don't lose the motivation to be with them, which does happen very quickly. I realized that devices can never help me manage my autistic brain because they simply develop things I can already do well. My autism is what makes devices so easy for me to understand, and it's also what makes people so complicated.

47. What Are the Key Ways of Ensuring the Family Environment Is Functional?

At the SACCADE Centre D'Expertise en Autisme, we have defined three keys to ensuring the family environment functions well. Here they are:

1. Recognize the signs of autism in your child for what they are, and don't confuse them with behavioural issues. The more you understand autism and the meaning of its manifestations, the easier it will be for you to work with these phenomena and help your child develop.
2. Understand the particularities of the autistic brain so that you can communicate better and feel competent. Once you figure out your child's way of communicating, your role as parent will be easier.
3. Understanding how autistic people experience emotions is essential for working with them and supporting children's relational development.

48. What Activities Should We As Parents Prioritize?

➤ **Myth: You cannot do activities with your child.**

Not true! Many activities can meet the needs of autistic people. Three concrete examples: swimming, cycling, and picture books. If the child can play a musical instrument, this will also be a very helpful activity.

Having access to a swimming pool has enormous benefits for an autistic person. You should choose times when there aren't many people so it's fairly quiet, and don't talk much to the child, to allow him to get the greatest benefit from the water.

Cycling is enriching for an autistic person because it also engages perceptive function.

Picture books should be available to the child at all times. Later, at the appropriate developmental stage, they should have access to graphic novels and dictionaries. Autistic children should be exposed early to books of all sorts.

49. What Is "Mild" Autism?

"She isn't autistic, she's just badly brought up!"

No, she hasn't been badly brought up, she is on the autism spectrum! Many parents have been shouted at and told that their child has been badly brought up and that they don't discipline her properly. Some people tell us that their child has mild autism. What does that actually mean? That the child isn't really on the autism spectrum?

Or that she has autism but it isn't visible? Or that it's so invisible that nothing can be done to help? And mild autism in relation to what?

The scientific literature confirms that autism is a condition. We need to look after this condition, just as a person with diabetes pays attention to their condition, whether they are mildly diabetic or otherwise.

If we think non-visible autism is mild and everything will be fine, we are making a mistake. If we think this means there is no point worrying about it or trying to intervene, we are making a mistake. As soon as we know that a person has ASD, we need to understand that there is work to be done. The individual needs help quickly to learn to rebalance herself in order to avoiding living out of sync with the world.

When a diagnosis of deafness is made, we immediately spring into action, coming up with action plans to ensure optimal development. But following a diagnosis of ASD, we generally wait for the symptoms to become obvious to everyone before helping the person. Why are we waiting?

50. Is It a Bad Thing If I Don't Consult All the Available Specialists About My Child?

No. The important thing is not mobilizing an entire team, but choosing a treatment that meets the person's needs and brings results. We thought for a long time that offering all kinds of therapies would necessarily ensure the development of the autistic person. But since the particular needs

> *Brigitte:* I had an elderly great-uncle, Uncle Charles, who used to say to me that if I wanted to grow carrots, I mustn't pull on their tops to make them grow faster. Why don't we heed this wise advice when it comes to autistic people? It's human development. Why do people try to pull them up instead of nurturing them so that they develop? Are we in such a hurry that it's worth ruining their lives? Encouragement from a young age means starting early, not trying to do everything!

of the autistic brain are not well known, therapies that make a real difference are rare.

It's vital to ask questions so you don't end up in treatment for life. You should ask questions like "When will we know if the work is done? What results will we see relative to the developmental stages of autism?"

It's important to respect the individual's stage of development. The expectations and learning need to be tailored to that stage. Ask yourself: Should I ask a child whose development is behind age level to do this?

51. Is There a Medication to Alleviate Autism?

At this time, no. However, many autistic people take medication for other reasons, for example hyperactivity, anxiety, sleep problems, etc. Some autistic people also take medication to reduce "problem behaviour" — if no help is given to support the autistic brain, the human body will keep trying unsuccessfully to re-establish internal equilibrium, a conflict that will be interpreted by others as behavioural problems.

Experience has shown us that medication has its limits when it comes to autism. At some point the real problem must be addressed, that is, controlling the autistic brain, with interventions adapted to autistic people rather than neurotypical people. When we pay attention to the autistic brain, the need for medication can often be reviewed with the doctor.

> We need to be careful with medication. Any treatment that isn't improving the situation should be reconsidered and changed. It's not helpful, whether or not a child has autism, to keep him on medication for months if it is not having any effect.

52. Can You Cure Autism?

➤ **Myth: There is a cure for autism!**

Unfortunately, people still continue to claim that they have cured their child.

Autism can't be cured. Since it's a difference in the way the brain is wired, it's part of the individual and their identity, just as deafness or blindness is part of a deaf or blind person.

Autistic manifestations (stimming and other typical behaviours) indicate the individual's stage of development. What proof is there of this? When autistic individuals are forced to suppress their movements, or when people try to make them pseudo-neurotypical, we notice three main autistic traits: difficulties with initiative, abstraction, and recalling

> Autism is not an illness and can't be "treated" with medica-
> tion. Other problems might require medication. Above all, we
> need to support the management of the autistic brain.

information in real time. Very often, people who believe
they have cured autism have simply smothered its most visible manifestations without concern for their purpose.

Autism is surrounded by myths that try to twist the
idea of autism to meet neurotypical people's needs. When
people talk about curing autism, who is really being helped
— the autistic person or the speaker? It's an important
question. Today, we accept that autism is a neurodevelopmental disorder; the disappearance of visible manifestations does not mean the autism is "cured."

> We need to qualify the statement that autism can't be
> cured. At this point, there is nothing that can "cure" autism.
> First of all, it's a neurodevelopmental disorder, not an illness.
> Next, not only is autism physiological, in the sense that it
> involves the brain's plasticity, it's also psychological, since its
> presence is part of a person's identity.
>
> Two powerful competing trends have emerged: the
> desire to make autistic gestures disappear and turn autis-
> tic individuals into pseudo-neurotypical people, believing
> them to be cured, and to demand rights for autistic people,
> defending neurodiversity and difference. But when we reach
> the point of being able to re-establish cerebral plasticity in
> autistic people, what will happen to that identity? This is a
> warning for everyone: we need to be humble, because this
> is an incredibly complex problem.

Brigitte: Autism is not something we have: it's what we are. It's part of our identity. What are we supposed to be cured of? Ourselves?

53. Why Do Autistic People Lack Initiative?

Everyone agrees that autistic people can do many things and have significant abilities. But people often wonder why it's so often necessary to take the initiative with the autistic person, to ask something specific of them so that they can act. He's intelligent, he can communicate, and he does the task well if we show him every time what needs to be done. Why can't he do this for himself? Even if we repeat the verbal instructions several times, he doesn't retain them. Is he lazy? Unmotivated?

The way the autistic brain is wired causes problems with initiative for all autistic people; this is one of the three characteristics of autism we have identified. We find this problem in the most severely affected autistic people, who can't re-establish equilibrium without help if their environment is disturbed. It also affects those who seem unable to get started, who seem to have an intellectual disability. These people always wait for clues before starting a task.

We find aspects of the same problem among many individuals — adults who have two or three degrees, but who can't live independently or hold down a job. The only difference in these two situations is the degree of severity of the autism.

We now know that it's possible to help them overcome this difficulty by working with them on cognitive organization, for example, by using SCL.

54. Every Time I Tidy Her Room and Put Away the Things That Are All Over the Place, She's Unhappy and Puts Everything Back Her Way. I Think It Was Better My Way.

➤ **Myth: For an autistic person, nothing can be moved, everything has to stay in the same place.**

An autistic adult might be used to putting his coat on the second hook in the hallway. When his mother comes over to help with the housework while he's out, she puts the coat in a different place, hanging it on the fourth hook instead, thinking she's doing the right thing. When the man notices, all hell breaks loose, and the mother doesn't understand why.

For autistic people, contextual meaning comes from what they see with their eyes in their environment. This environment needs to stay unchanged to maintain the same meaning. Just as some people can't work unless papers are strewn all over their desk, an autistic person can't make sense of his environment if it's been changed, or not until he has moved through all the necessary developmental stages. Tidying and putting the papers in order helps the person to start thinking about work; the work of putting the papers in order corresponds to the necessary development of the cognitive structure. To encourage him, go ahead with any changes in the individual's presence, with his help, never in his absence. That way he can reconfigure his environment in real time.

An autistic person isn't just obstinately refusing to do what he is asked. His insistence comes from his brain's need to figure out the meaning of his surroundings.

55. What Support Can the Extended Family (Grandparents, Aunts, Uncles, etc.) Give?

First of all, members of the extended family must understand what autism is: they need to understand before judging. They must not fall into the trap of misinterpreting what might seem like behavioural problems but are actually problems with internal control.

Remember, when an autistic person moves her arms, or has a different idea about games or objects, or walks on tiptoe, these actions have meaning for her. She is responding

---

When you're with a person on the autism spectrum ...

- Slow down; give her time to get her bearings with you. The conversation will improve once she reaches certain developmental stages and possesses behaviour strategies that her brain can access more easily.
- Speak less when you are talking to her; this will allow her to understand what you expect.
- Speak more quietly in her presence; this will feel less disruptive to her.
- Situate actions in real time, in a simple and visual way, in her presence; for example, "Grandpa is with you, we're going to do a jigsaw, then we'll go for a walk, and then it will be time for dinner."
- Remember that autism is a neurodevelopmental disorder; do not insist that the child behave in a certain way in social situations just because it's age-appropriate. Allow her the time to learn at her own pace, even if she is very intelligent.

Brigitte: You can count on autistic people to quickly pick up on whether their movements and gestures bother you! We soon realize that we are unwelcome. Society is always asking autistic people to pass as neurotypical — in other words, not to disturb people. But this means that we are not responding to our own needs but to those of neurotypical people. When neurotypical people demand that we behave in a certain way, they aren't even interested in knowing if we're able to do it. But are our lives worth any less than theirs?

to a fundamental need, an internal command — the same thing that happens when we have hiccups.

The family can recognize that the autistic person has great potential but that he needs help, and that, very often, his behaviour expresses not aggression but confusion in the face of the perceived incoherence of the world around him.

The extended family is extremely valuable for parents of autistic children. Current research tells us that the family of an autistic person needs training to have a good chance of success in their efforts to help. The parents need to be capable of explaining to the extended family that they have a significant supportive role to play, whether that is supporting the child, supporting his siblings, or helping the parents find time to recharge their batteries.

CONCLUSION

Hope

Autistic people just want to be helped. The autistic individual has already started to help himself, and has been managing his situation from very early on, probably since birth, even if his autism was identified only later. So how can we continue to help?

- Respect the particular characteristics of his cognitive structure and autistic development.
- Respect her visual brain.
- Accept that his autism is not part-time.
- Accept that even though she can't do what other people do, she can do more than other people in certain areas.
- Accept that just loving him is not enough, because autism is not an emotional disorder.
- Understand that autism does not fade over time, that it's part and parcel of the person.
- Accept that she speaks another language, and that there's no point asking her to change how she communicates;

it's up to neurotypical people to communicate in other ways and meet her on her own terms.

- Understand that autism is a neurodevelopmental disorder and that it relates to a particular brain wiring that is not visible.
- Understand that an autistic person is more than just autistic.
- Learn about the reasons for different kinds of interventions, how long they take, and what results are anticipated. Children are not lab rats.
- Insist on a coordinated approach from specialists if several experts are involved. An autistic person is a human being!
- Be attentive. If the results are slow to come, or if you aren't comfortable with the treatment, quit!
- Be cautious around approaches, beliefs, and myths that send you down meaningless paths. You need to trust your instincts.

The most important thing is understanding how autism works. What are the repercussions for the individual of having an autistic brain, and how can the people around her help her to manage her own particular situation? Only autistic people can answer this question, because they alone can manage their own autism. But autistic individuals' brains are less adept at social communication, and those individuals are surrounded by people who do not have a way of communicating with them. So how can they make themselves understood and transmit their message to others?

Autism is a neurodevelopmental disorder and it can evolve. Experts need to take a neurodevelopmental approach, that is, an approach that helps brain development and therefore overall development. A positive intervention would work to develop brain initiative, facilitate access to abstract thinking, and reduce information-processing speeds. But as many parents have said, the best indicator of success remains the observation that talking to their child has become more natural — not because he is no longer on the autism spectrum, but because a bridge has been built between the individual and the people around him.

Brain plasticity affects development. Random or ill-conceived approaches run the risk of creating additional problems. Too many autistic people have ended up with an acquired intellectual delay or with behavioural problems, not because experts didn't make an effort or lacked good intentions, but because their knowledge was incomplete. You can't make up autism expertise as you go along: the consequences for the autistic person are too severe. We must always know why we are trying a particular approach.

When we try to modify one behaviour or make it disappear and others appear in its place, or the person becomes extremely upset, it's because the autistic brain structure itself has been disrupted. You need to trust the person: if she is screaming in distress, it's because the approach isn't working for her and she doesn't have the language to articulate her reaction. You can trust nature: if someone can't say something, they can still show it! It's cruel to leave an autistic person to cry, as if we were dealing with an object rather than a human being. We have come to believe that autism itself does less harm than social judgment and false beliefs.

Can we say that people need a certain kind of expert simply because they are on the autism spectrum? No. First of all we need to assess their needs and stop trying random approaches. Many autistic people are happy and making regular progress. It's not the degree of severity that dictates whether an autistic person is happy or not, but the stability of their cognitive structure.

We need to try to understand autism so that our efforts are appropriately targeted and address the needs of the person concerned: the autistic one. Autistic people's needs are very different from those of neurotypical people.

The origins of autism remain a mystery, but the workings of the autistic brain are becoming more accessible to us. Understanding these workings allows us to intervene much more effectively to improve social skills, reciprocal interactions, and social awareness. That way, many individuals can move away from memorized behaviour patterns and reach a much more spontaneous self-direction, regardless of the degree of severity of their autism. We now hear parents tell us that their child is affectionate, that she says "I love you" out loud or shows affection.

If the physiological and psychological issues around autism are complex, that is not the fault of the individual, but of the human brain, which is also highly complex. Based on clinical practice, history, and the literature, we have enough knowledge to know what needs to be done, but it can't be a one-size-fits-all approach. And we need to be careful not to repeat the errors of our predecessors. Many of them were brilliant scientists: if an approach did not work for them, it won't work for us either.

Now that we have developed SACCADE Conceptual Language, a specialized conceptual language, autistic people can communicate and learn, and above all have access to a certain quality of life. Social blindness won't be reduced by learning manners by rote or using apps, but by developing the ability to interact with real individuals. That is how human nature works.

About the Authors

Brigitte Harrisson

Brigitte Harrisson, a social worker, ASD expert, and autistic person, co-founded Concept ConsulTED Inc. in 2006, which has since become the SACCADE Centre D'Expertise en Autisme in Quebec. Since 2004, she has given hundreds of training sessions, workshops, and talks about autism for school boards, hospitals (psychiatry and child psychiatry), centres for health and social services, rehabilitation centres for people with intellectual disabilities and pervasive developmental disorders, daycare centres, and community organizations. Since 2003, she has presented her work to over 25,000 people, and has been cited by authors in countries around the world.

With over twenty years of experience in health and social services in Quebec and New Brunswick, Harrisson has worked as a specialist consultant for organizations working in the ASD field and taught the SACCADE model to young people with ASD. She also has many years' experience in family counselling and in counselling children and teens with ASD.

Harrisson has published articles in the magazines of Autisme Montréal, Autisme Alsace, FQATED (the Quebec association for ASD and PDD), Autisme Québec, and TED* Sans Frontières, and has given interviews with print and television media. She was president of SATEDI (the international francophone organization for autism and pervasive developmental disorders) for two years, and then the Canadian vice-president for several years. In 2006, she was invited to take part in the Standing Committee on Social Affairs, Science and Technology consultation on pervasive developmental disorders. She also took part in the National Autism Conference in Toronto in 2007.

Harrisson has worked closely with various committees, including steering RNETSA (Quebec's ASD expertise network), under the aegis of the Quebec Ministers for Health and Social Services and Education, Leisure, and Sport from 2006 to 2011. She was director at large at Autism Canada.

She took part in creating resources such as the DVDs *L'Autisme vu de l'intérieur* (Autism seen from the inside, 2004), produced by the Centre de Communication en Santé Mentale (CECOM) of Rivière-des-Prairies Hospital, and *Déficience intellectuelle et troubles envahissants du développement* (Intellectual disability and pervasive developmental disorders), produced by the Department of Health and Social Services in collaboration with Laval University, which provides a training tool for health and social services centres and intellectual disability services in

---

* TED = *troubles envahissants du développement*, i.e., pervasive development ment disorder, or PDD.

Quebec. She also took part in the special autism edition of *Québec Science* magazine in April 2015.

Lise St-Charles

Co-founder of Concept ConsulTED Inc., and later of the SACCADE Centre D'Expertise en Autisme, Lise St-Charles has a DESS in ASD intervention supervision. She has also taught courses at the University of Montreal and Laval University in the certificate and degree programs for treatment of pervasive developmental disorders.

She worked for several years in Dr. Guy Rouleau's team at CHUM (the University of Montreal Health Centre), researching the relationship between genetics and autism; she has more than thirty years' experience in one of Quebec's CRDITED rehabilitation centres, primarily working with children, teens, and adults with ASD and their families, supervising the intensive behavioural intervention program for children aged five and under, and working as a clinical ASD specialist for five- to ninety-nine-year-olds. She works closely with the medical fields of psychiatry and child psychiatry in ASD assessment. She is also the designer and author of the regional services plan "Un réseau de services aux personnes présentant un trouble envahissant du développement et à leur famille" (A network of integrated services for people with pervasive developmental disorders and their families, 2001), which was adopted by the regional health and social services board in the Bas-Saint-Laurent region. In 2002, she was part of the national advisory committee for the action plan on services for people with pervasive developmental disorders and their families. From 2001 to 2007 she was a member of the business affairs committee of the Quebec federation of CRDI (the Centre for Rehabilitation of Intellectual Disabilities), working on skills development for people with pervasive developmental disorders (PDD). She helped create a needs assessment as a member of the training subcommittee of the special working group of PDD experts as part of the national PDD training plan (2003–2007).

St-Charles has led training sessions in several teaching institutions at a national and international level. She was an early collaborator with the Mira Foundation in 2002, in the provincial pilot project providing dogs for children with ASD, and from 2002 to 2007 she was also clinical director of "family fresh air" summer camps for children, teens, and adults with ASD. She has been active in the autism field for more than forty years and follows with interest new developments in the field of ASD intervention. The many programs, approaches, and tools used over the decades, such as TEACCH, PECS, social stories, and ABA, among others, are very familiar to her: she has hundreds of hours of training on every aspect of autism, based on everything that has been presented in Quebec over the past forty years, from Brenda Myles to Barry Prizant, by way of Steven Gutstein, Tony Charman, Pamela Wolfberg, Mark L. Sundberg, J. D. Dougherty, and Carol Gray.

The SACCADE Partnership

Brigitte Harrisson and Lise St-Charles are co-authors of the SACCADE model.

They teach courses in the ASD certificate program at the University of Quebec at Rimouski, a program they helped to create. They have also taught at the University of Montreal and Laval University. Their published articles include "Hypothèse du fonctionnement interne de la structure de pensée" (Hypothesis of the internal function of thought structure) in *Psychologie & éducation* (June 2012) and "La structure de pensée autistique et la scolarisation" (Autistic thought structure and education) in *La nouvelle revue de l'adaptation et de la scolarisation* (January 2013). Together, they have addressed teams in the medical world as well as the AQETA (the institute for learning disabilities in Quebec), the APEESQ (the association for special education teachers of Quebec), the Montreal teachers' union, Autisme France, Autisme Suisse Romande, and the Salon de l'autisme.

Brigitte Harrisson and Lise St-Charles have collaborated on pilot treatment projects with institutions such as specialist schools, daycares, and centres for people with intellectual disabilities. They regularly offer training sessions across Canada and in other countries, such as Switzerland and France (in Lorraine and Martinique), where they work in collaboration with various autism organizations.

In 2016 they were named the Le Soleil/Radio-Canada Laureates in the "society" category for founding the SACCADE Centre D'Expertise en Autisme.

Bibliography

American Psychiatric Association. *Diagnostics and Statistical Manual of Mental Disorders (DSM-5)*, fifth edition, 2013.

Baron-Cohen, Simon. *Mindblindness: An Essay on Autism and Theory of Mind*, MIT Press, 1995.

Brossard, Michel. "Lev Vygotski. Le rôle des interactions," *Les grands dossiers des sciences humaines — Les grands penseurs de l'éducation*, December 2016/January – February 2017; 45: 50–51.

Brosseau, Cynthia. "Autisme et attachement dans la famille," *Intervention*, 2008; 129; 69–78.

Chamak, B. "Les récits de personnes autistes : une analyse socio-anthropologique," *Handicap — Revue de sciences humaines et sociales*, 2005; 105–6: 33–50.

Costand, G. "Détection d'un gène commun à l'autisme et à l'épilepsie," *L'Actualité médicale*, 8 June 2011, 22.

Courchesne, E. et al. "Mapping early brain development in autism," *Neuron*, 2007; 56(2): 399–413.

Duclos, G. *L'Estime de soi, un passeport pour la vie*, Montréal, Éditions du CHU Sainte-Justine, 2004.

Fassio, A. et al. "SYN1 loss-of-function mutations in autism and partial epilepsy cause impaired synaptic function," *Human Molecular Genetics*, 2011; 20(12): 2297–307.

Frith, Uta. *Autism: Explaining the Enigma*, Wiley-Blackwell, 2003.

Grandin, Temple. *Thinking in Pictures: My Life With Autism*, Vintage, 2006.

Grandin, Temple. *Temple Talks … About Autism and Sensory Issues*, Sensory World, 2015.

Harrisson, Brigitte, with Lise St-Charles. *L'Autisme: au-delà des apparences*, Rivière-du-Loup, Éditions Concept ConsulTED, 2010.

Hochman, Jacques. *Histoire de l'autisme*, Paris, Odile Jacob, 2009.

Jalinière, Hugo. "Autisme: d'où vient leur hypersensibilité?" sciencesetavenir.fr/sante/20140515.OBS7323/autisme-d-ou-vient-leur-hypersensibilite.html.

Jordan, R., & S. Powell. *Understanding and Teaching Children with Autism*, Wiley, 1995.

Just, M.A. et al. "Cortical activation and synchronization during sentence comprehension in high-functioning autism: Evidence of underconnectivity," *Brain*, 2004; 127(8): 1811–21.

Lestienne, Rémy. *Le Cerveau cognitif*, Paris, CNRS Éditions, 2016.

Mottron, Laurent. *L'Autisme, une autre intelligence*, Bruxelles, Mardaga, 2004.

Mottron, Laurent. *L'Intervention précoce pour enfants autistes*, Bruxelles, Mardaga, 2016.

Ozonoff, S., B. F. Pennington, & S. Rogers. "Executive function deficits in high-functioning autistic individuals: Relationship of theory of mind," *Journal of Child Psychology and Psychiatry*, 1991; 32(7): 1081–105.

Philip, Christine. *Autisme et parentalité*, Paris, Dunod, 2009.

Poirier, N., and C. Des Rivières-Pigeon. *Le Trouble du spectre autistique: État des connaissances*, Presses de l'Université du Québec, 2013.

Radio-Canada. "Les écrans, ces ennemis du sommeil," interview with Véronique Daneau of the Centre de santé du sommeil de l'Hôpital Sacré-Coeur (Montréal), ici.radio-canada.ca/emissions/la_sphere/2015-2016/ chronique.asp?idChronique=387405.

Vermeulen, Peter. *Autism as Context Blindness*, Shawnee (KS), AAPC Publishing, 2012.

Vermeulen, Peter. *Autisme et émotions*, Leuven, De Boeck, 2009. Originally published as *Een gesloten boek. Autisme en emoties*, Leuven, Acco, 2000.

Vermeulen, Peter. *Comprendre les personnes autistes de haut niveau*, Paris, Dunod, 2009. Originally published as *Brein bedriegt. Als Autisme niet op autisme lijkt* (1998), Berchem, EPO Uitgeverij, 2009.

Williams, Donna. *Nobody Nowhere*, Jessica Kingsley Publishers, 1998. Originally published in 1992 by Doubleday.

Glossary

autism spectrum disorders: Autism is now generally called autism spectrum disorder (ASD). This term applies to autistic people as well as those affected by Asperger's or unspecified pervasive developmental disorders (PDD).

behavioural problems: Inappropriate ways of acting and reacting. These include negative, hostile, and provocative behaviours.

cognitive organization work: Modifying the brain's wiring with the goal of changing the cognitive processes. Depending on the desired outcome, cognitive remediation work can focus on equilibrium and neural synchronization to improve an individual's ability to categorize information; to make links, analogies, and deductions; and to analyze or reason.

cognitive organization: The way in which all mental operations work together to facilitate information processing.

developmental stage: One of the major physical, psychological, and cognitive human developmental stages defined by neuroscience and psychology.

dynamic: Characterized by movement and progress in brain development (as opposed to static).

homeostasis: A fundamental biological characteristic of the human body, which tries to maintain a stable internal environment by mitigating the effects of disequilibrium. Since the body is in a constantly changing environment, it reacts by constantly adjusting to minimize the effects of these changes and return to its initial state or a new stable state.

inflexible: Demonstrating significant intransigence, applying the letter of the law, and exhibiting behaviour characterized by a lack of flexibility.

information processing: A specific cognitive process by which information captured by the brain is transformed into mental operations.

low processing speed: Speed at which the various mental operations are initiated and executed — slower than in neurotypical individuals.

neural equilibrium: Consistent transmission across the neural networks of the different areas of the brain, leading to a state of stability and harmony.

neurodevelopmental disorder: A neurological problem apparent early in life in which the brain's wiring affects the individual's development.

neurotypical: A person who is not on the autism spectrum.

over-connection: An increased number of connections between neurons in some areas of the brain.

Information transmission in these areas of the brain is quicker and more significant than usual.

plasticity: The brain's ability to alter connections in the neural networks based on its experiences.

proprioception: The perception, whether conscious or not, of the position of the various parts of the body.

SCL (SACCADE Conceptual Language): Created by Brigitte Harrisson and Lise St-Charles, SCL is a proprietary written code based on the harmonization of concepts and of the spoken language as a reference language. It allows communication to be established between autistic people and neurotypical people, and thus can be used as a bridge between people with differently wired brains. SCL comprises conceptual tools and practical applications. SCL is not yet available in English.

self-stimulation (stimming): Repetitive movements that seem to have no apparent purpose. Often observed in children with developmental disorders, stimming can have various causes, including seeking sensory stimulation or reducing the effect of overstimulation.

sensory integration: The process by which the brain integrates and organizes sensory experiences such as touch, smell, taste, hearing, and proprioception. Children need this base to be able to later access more complex learning and behaviour structures.

sensory processing disorder: Difficulty interpreting the type and intensity of incoming sensory information.

static: Something with little or no movement or no fluidity, something that does not evolve or stays fixed (as opposed to dynamic).

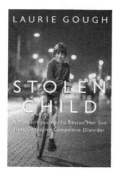

STOLEN CHILD
A Mother's Journey to Rescue Her
Son from Obsessive Compulsive
Disorder
LAURIE GOUGH

**A year in the desperate life of a boy transformed
by OCD from a bright ten-year-old into a
stranger in his own skin.**

Although Laurie Gough was an intrepid traveller who had explored wild, far-off reaches of the globe, the journey she and her family took in their own home in their small Quebec village proved to be far more frightening, strange, and foreign than any land she had ever visited.

It began when Gough's son, shattered by his grandfather's death, transformed from a bright, soccer-ball kicking ten-year-old into a near-stranger, falling into trances where his parents couldn't reach him and performing ever-changing rituals of magical thinking designed to bring his grandpa back to life.

Stolen Child examines a horrifying year in one family's life, the lengths the parents went to to help their son, and how they won the battle against his all-consuming disorder.

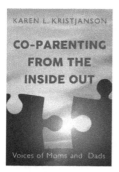

CO-PARENTING FROM THE INSIDE OUT
Voices of Moms and Dads
KAREN L. KRISTJANSON
FOREWORD BY EDWARD KRUK

Karen L. Kristjanson shares the stories of a variety of divorced and separated couples who co-parent.

Effective co-parenting, or sharing significant parenting time with an ex-spouse, is one of the best gifts separated parents can give to their children. The interviews in *Co-Parenting from the Inside Out* are with real moms and dads in diverse circumstances, showing them making choices, sometimes struggling, and often growing. Their stories offer insights into wise decision-making, as well as practical strategies that strengthen families. Parents can see that they are not alone as they navigate their feelings and build a future. While pain exists in most stories, there is also hope. Co-parents often feel that they have become more confident and compassionate, and parent better than before. The effects of their personal growth and their children's are the silver lining in the dark pain of divorce.

Karen L. Kristjanson has brought together real life co-parenting stories that inspire separated parents and help them understand co-parenting better, offering practical tips and tools that directly benefit families.

Book Credits

Project Editors: Kathryn Lane and Elena Radic
Editor: Claire Wilkshire
Proofreader: Emma Warnken Johnson

Designer: Laura Boyle

Publicist: Elham Ali

Dundurn

Publisher: J. Kirk Howard
Vice-President: Carl A. Brand
Editorial Director: Kathryn Lane
Artistic Director: Laura Boyle
Production Manager: Rudi Garcia
Manager, Accounting and Technical Services: Livio Copetti

Editorial: Allison Hirst, Dominic Farrell, Jenny McWha,
Rachel Spence, Elena Radic, Melissa Kawaguchi

Marketing and Publicity: Kendra Martin, Elham Ali,
Heather McLeod

Design and Production: Sophie Paas-Lang

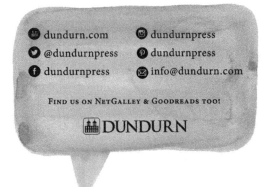

dundurn.com
@dundurnpress
dundurnpress

dundurnpress
dundurnpress
info@dundurn.com

FIND US ON NETGALLEY & GOODREADS TOO!

DUNDURN